MEET INNER FIT GIRL, YOUR FITNESS CHAMPION!

SHE'S THAT LITTLE VOICE INSIDE THAT TELLS YOU TO EXERCISE—TAKE THE STAIRS INSTEAD OF THE ELEVATOR OR TAKE A WALK BEFORE YOU WATCH TV, ETC.

HER GOAL IS TO HELP EVERYONE GET THEIR RECOMMENDED 150 MINUTES OF EXERCISE EACH WEEK. WHILE SOME PEOPLE DO TAKE HER ADVICE, MANY MORE DON'T. INSTEAD, THEY OFFER UP ALL KINDS OF EXCUSES.

THIS BOOK IS A LIST OF THOSE EXCUSES, 100 TOTAL, ALONG WITH INNER FIT GIRL'S IDEAS FOR BEATING THESE EXCUSES!

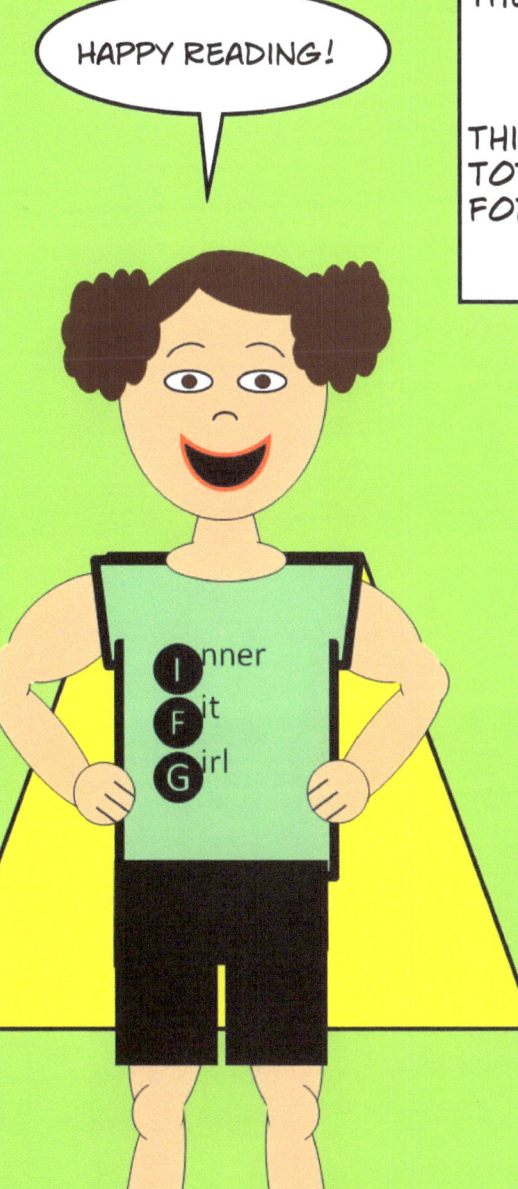

HAPPY READING!

© 2014 Noelle Allen

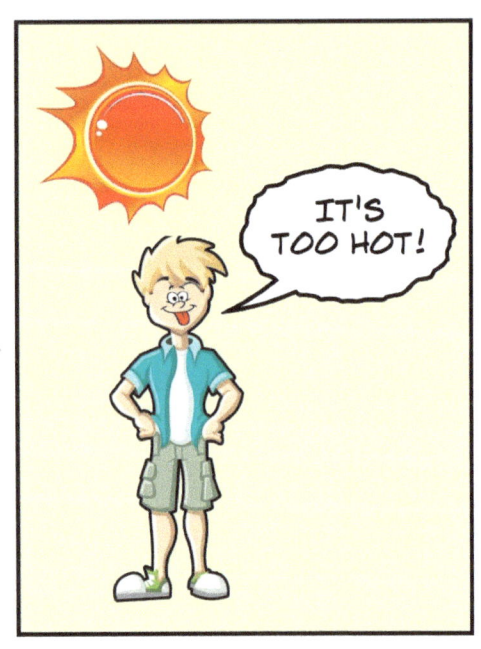

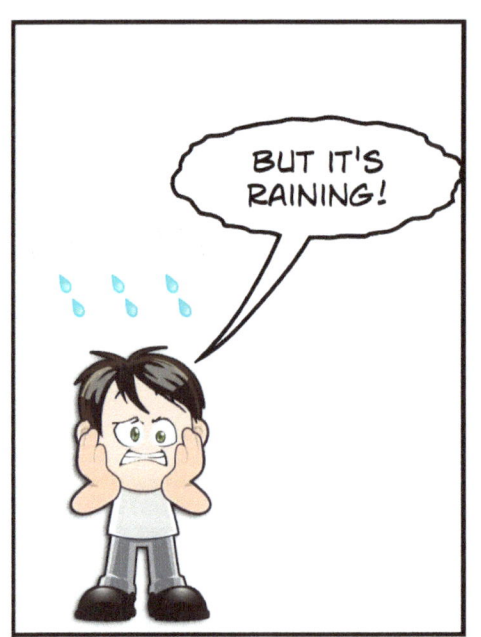

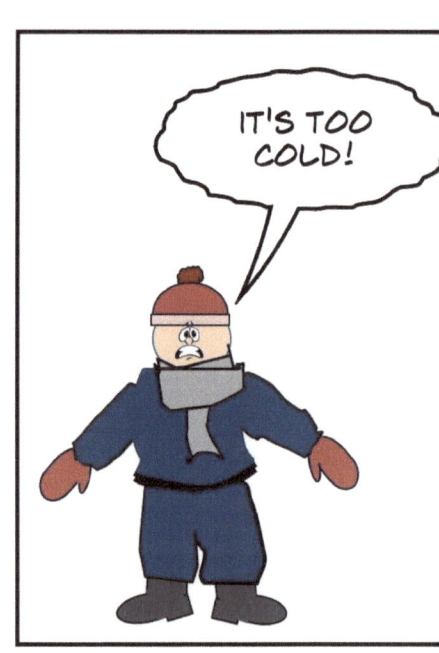

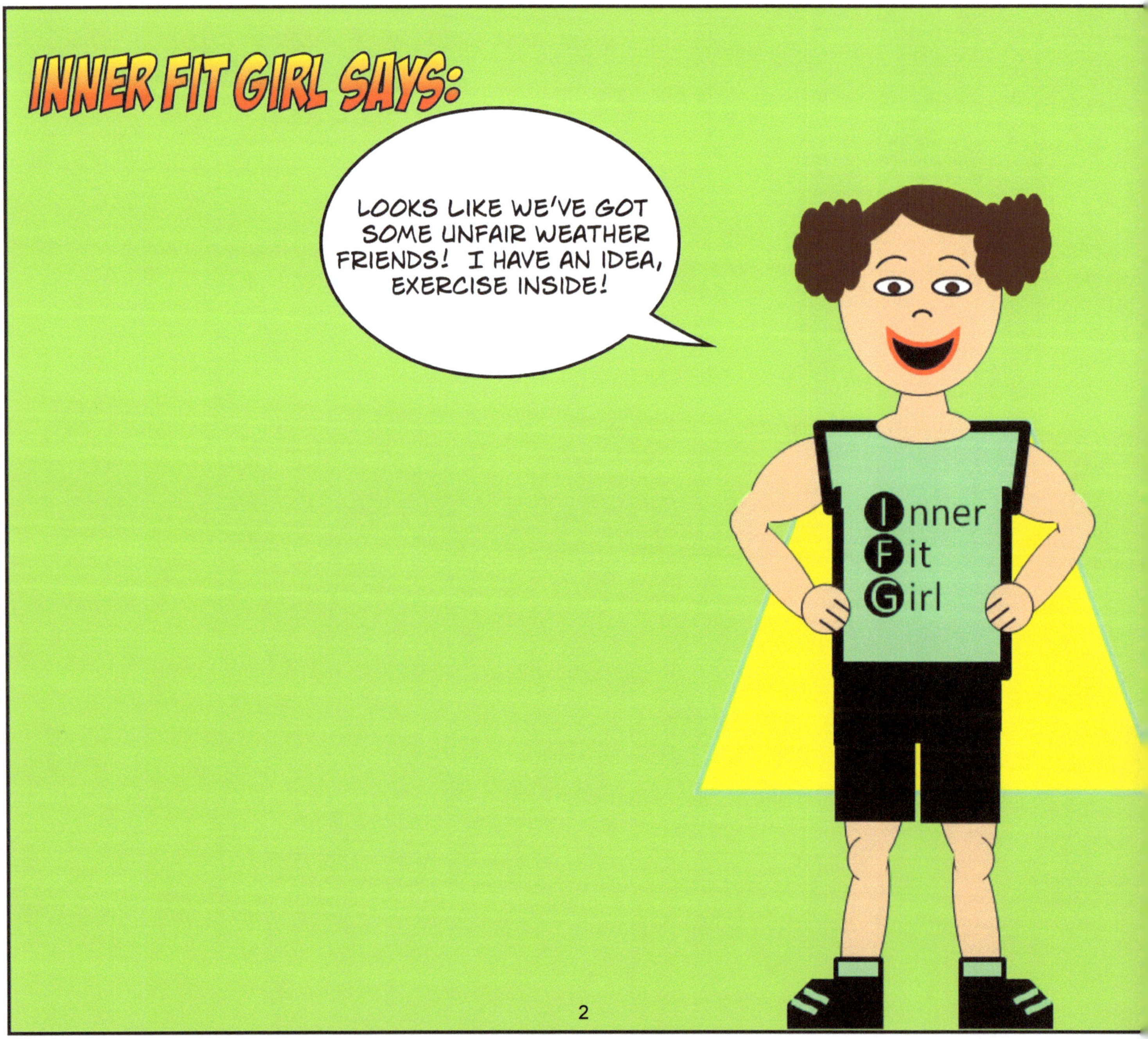

INNER FIT GIRL SAYS:

LOOKS LIKE WE'VE GOT SOME UNFAIR WEATHER FRIENDS! I HAVE AN IDEA, EXERCISE INSIDE!

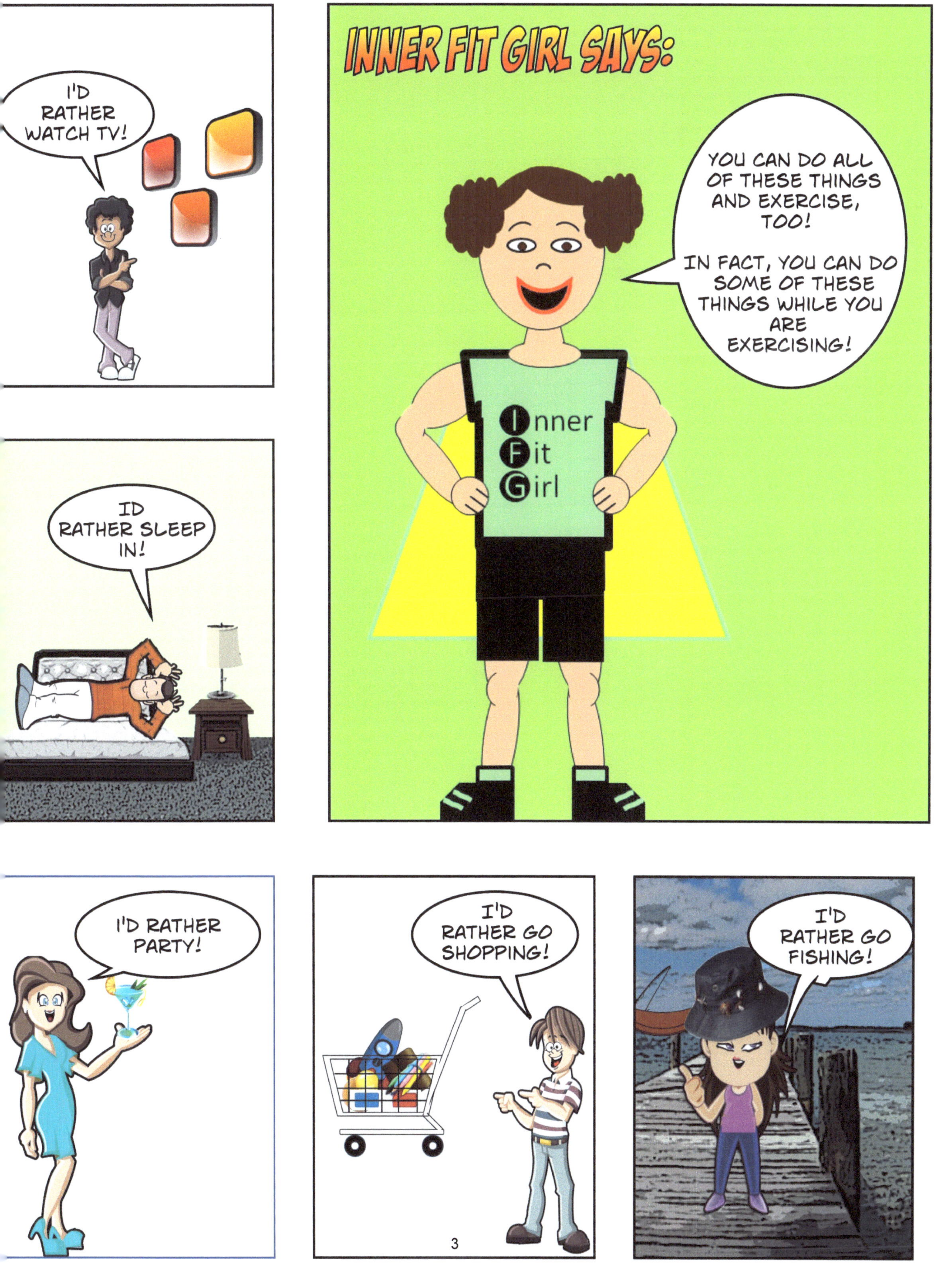

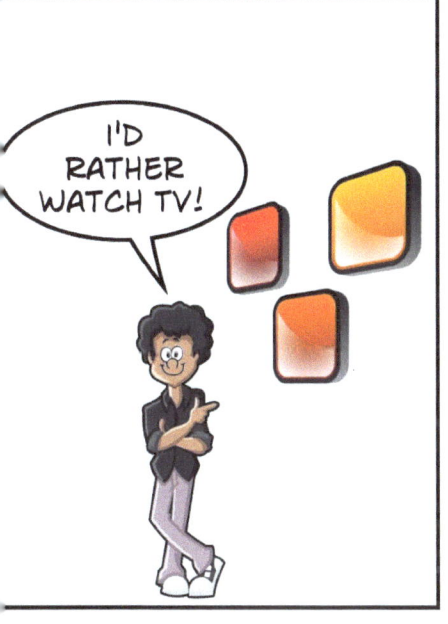

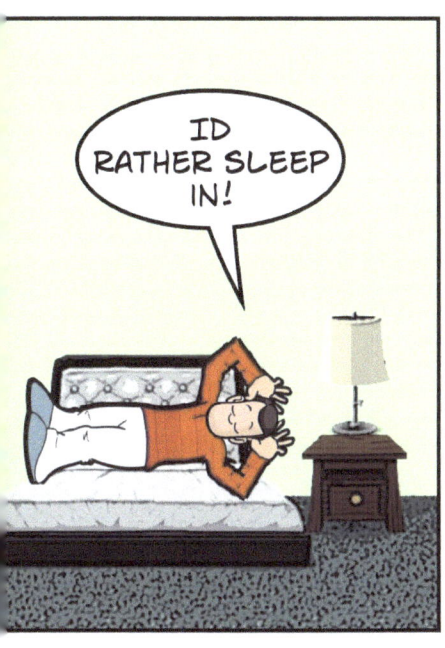

INNER FIT GIRL SAYS:

YOU CAN DO ALL OF THESE THINGS AND EXERCISE, TOO!

IN FACT, YOU CAN DO SOME OF THESE THINGS WHILE YOU ARE EXERCISING!

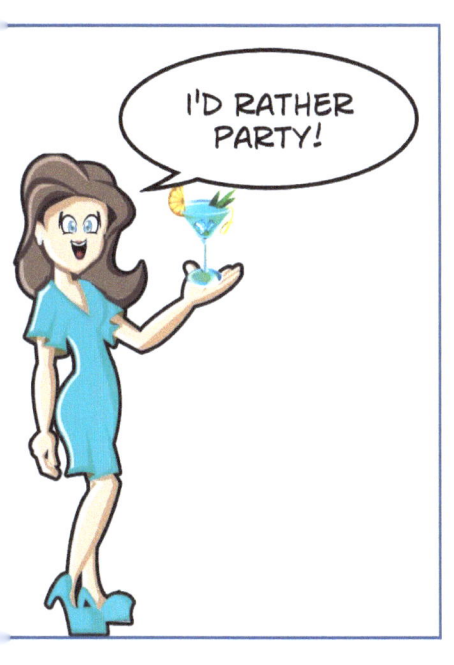

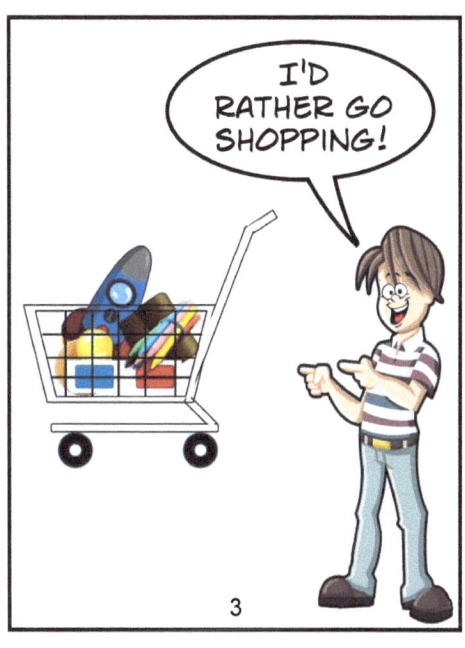

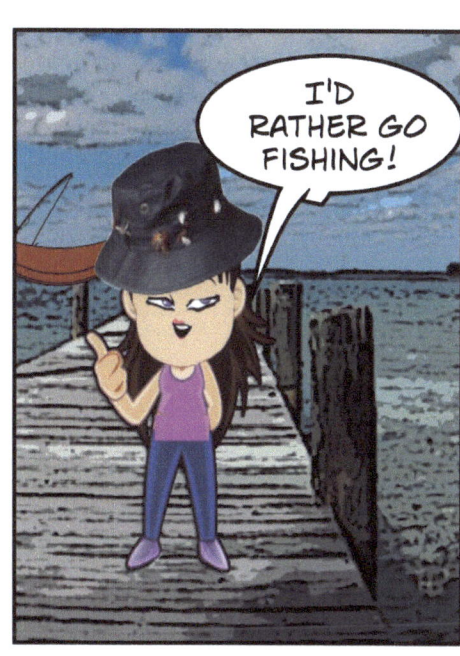

3

GYM MEMBERSHIP IS TOO EXPENSIVE!

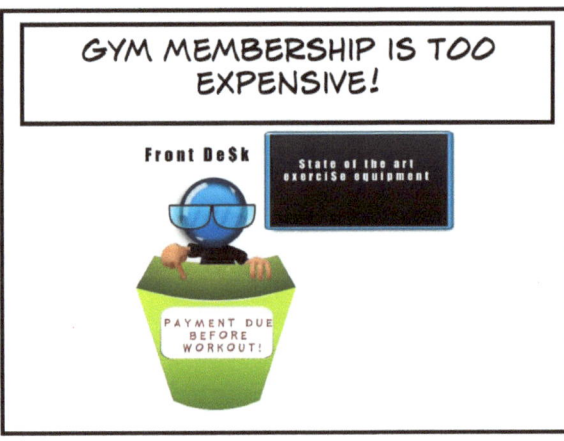

I CAN'T AFFORD A PERSONAL TRAINER!

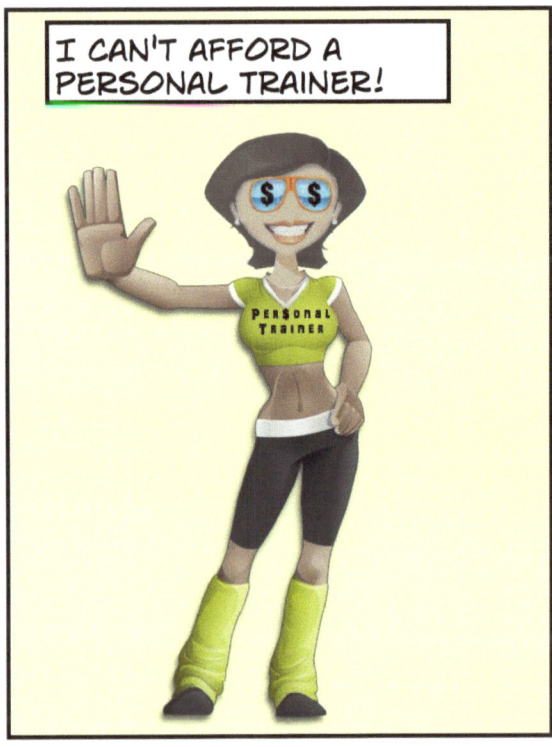

HOME EXERCISE EQUIPMENT COSTS TOO MUCH!

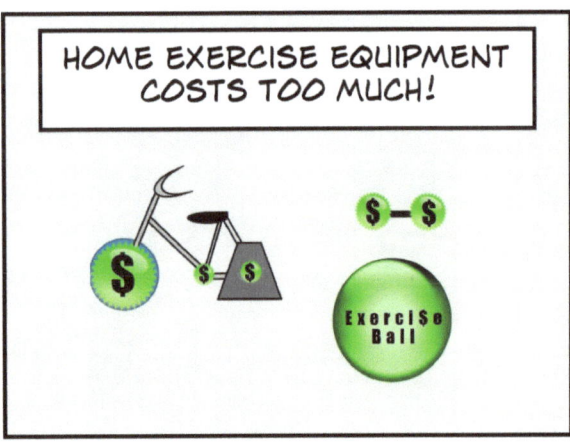

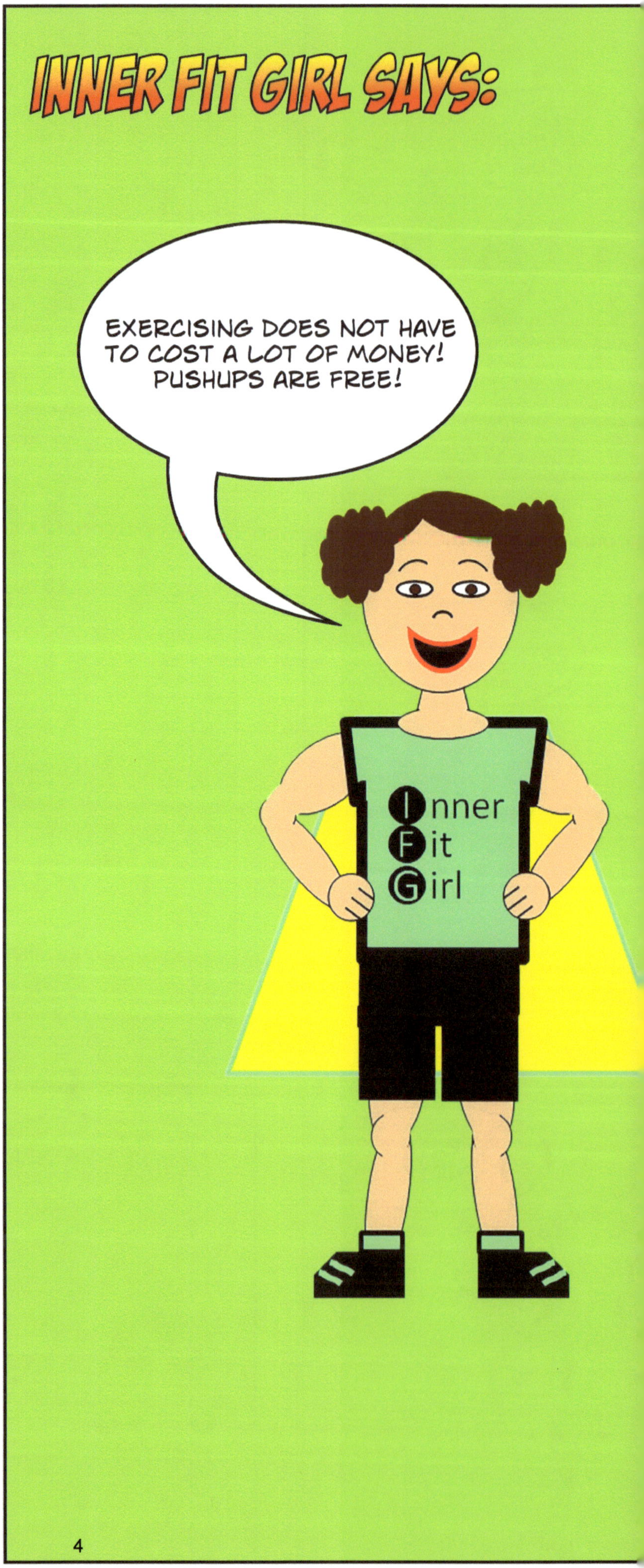

INNER FIT GIRL SAYS:

EXERCISING DOES NOT HAVE TO COST A LOT OF MONEY! PUSHUPS ARE FREE!

4

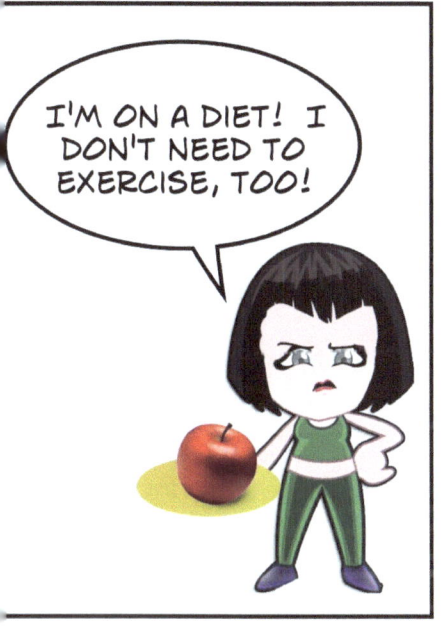

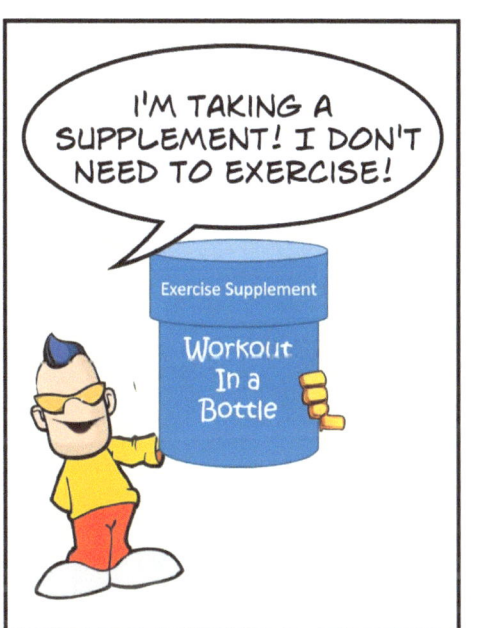

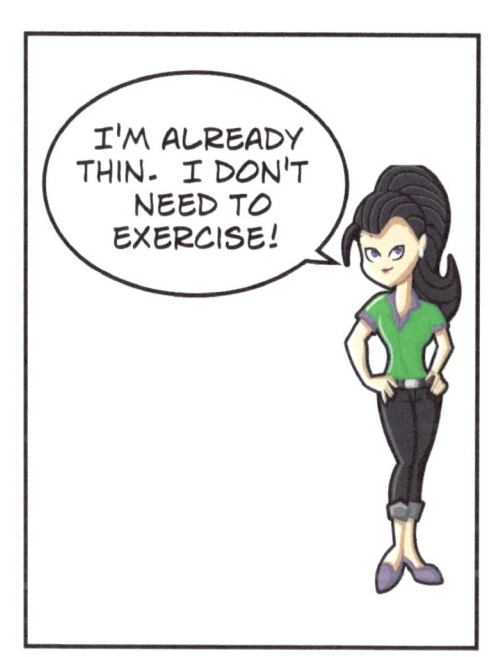

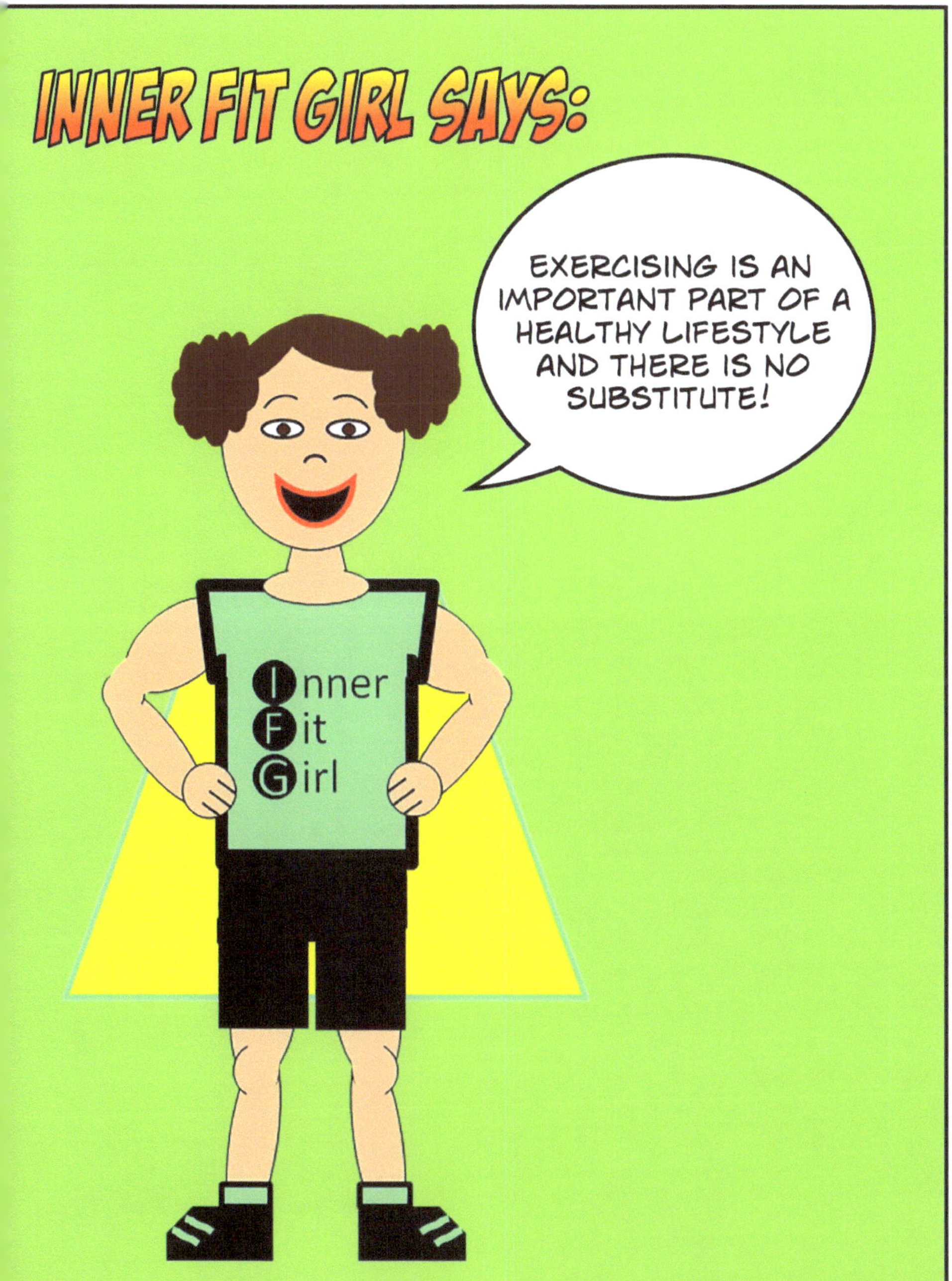

INNER FIT GIRL SAYS:

EXERCISING IS AN IMPORTANT PART OF A HEALTHY LIFESTYLE AND THERE IS NO SUBSTITUTE!

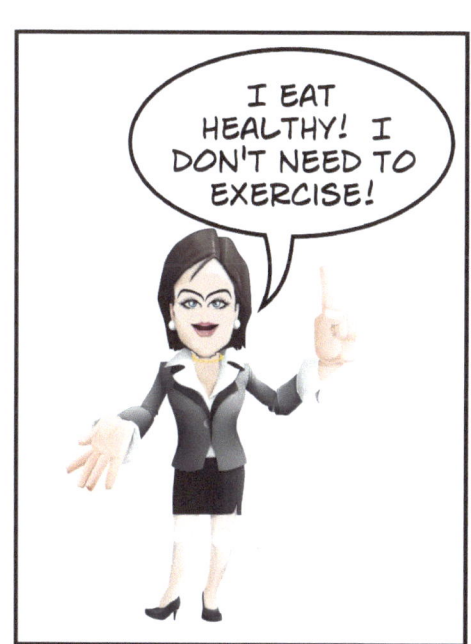

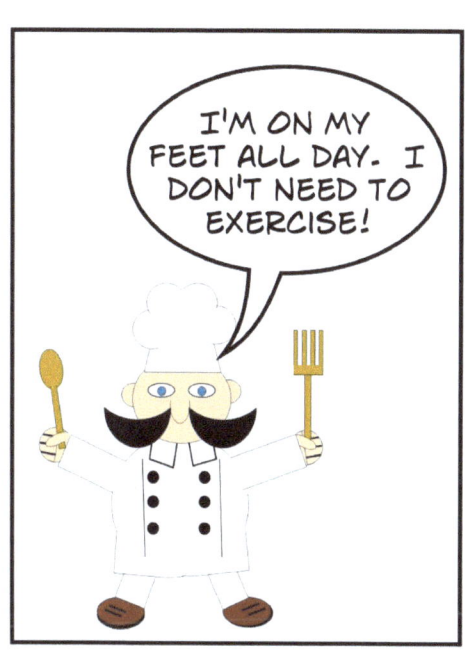

5

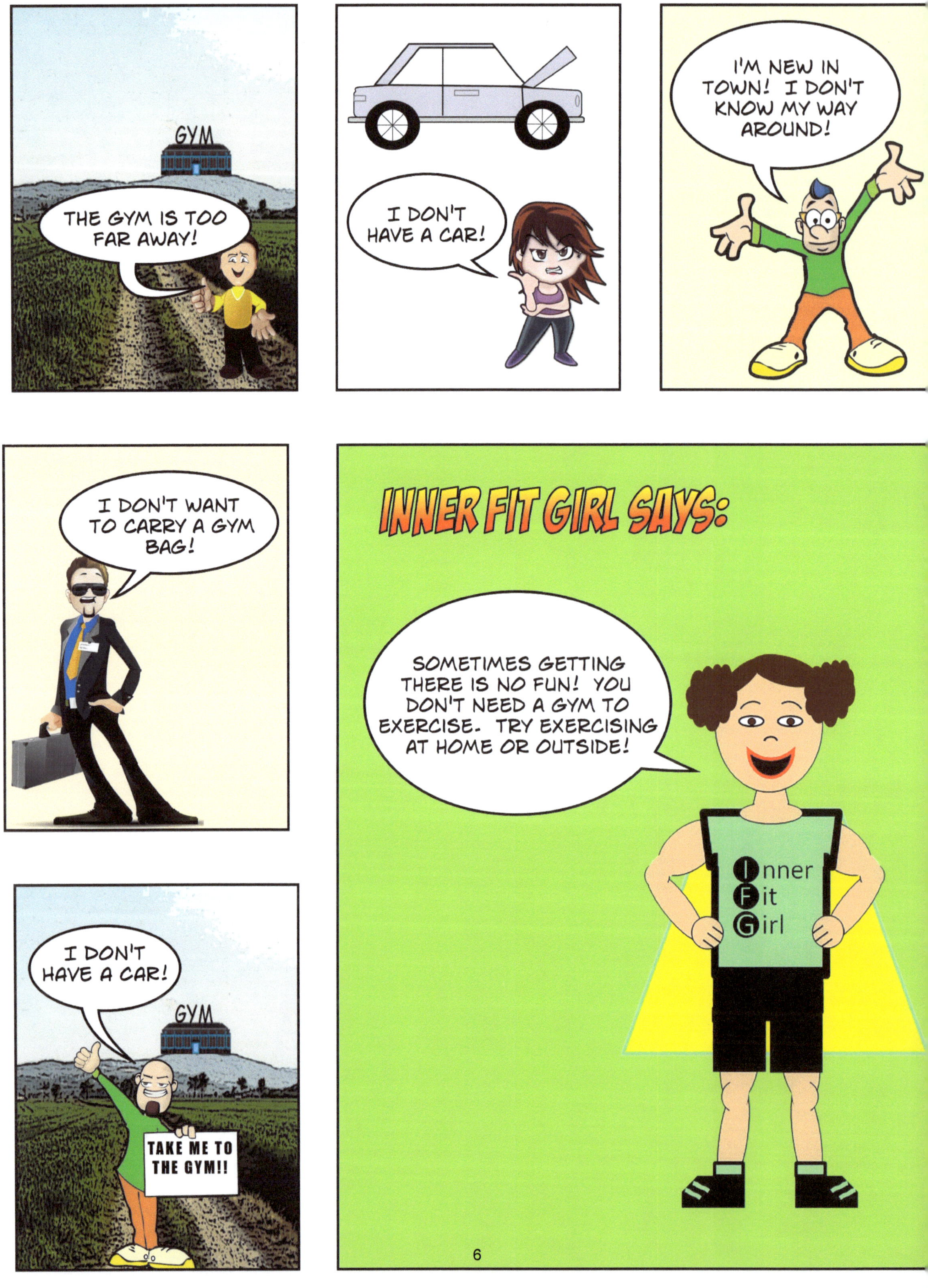

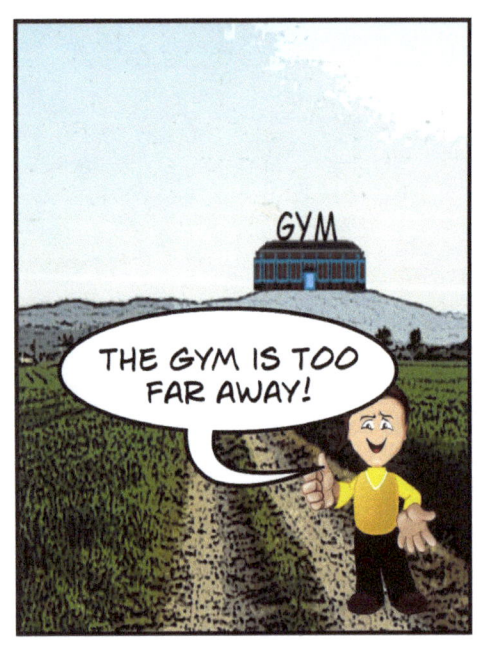

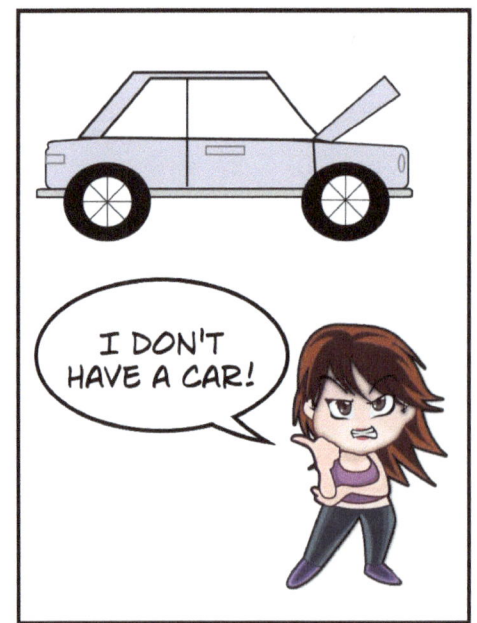

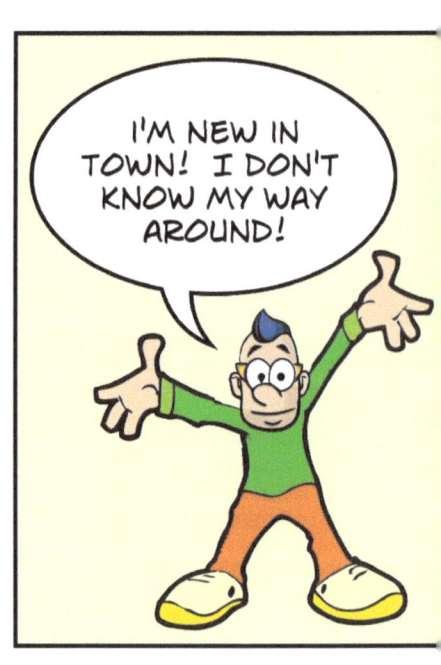

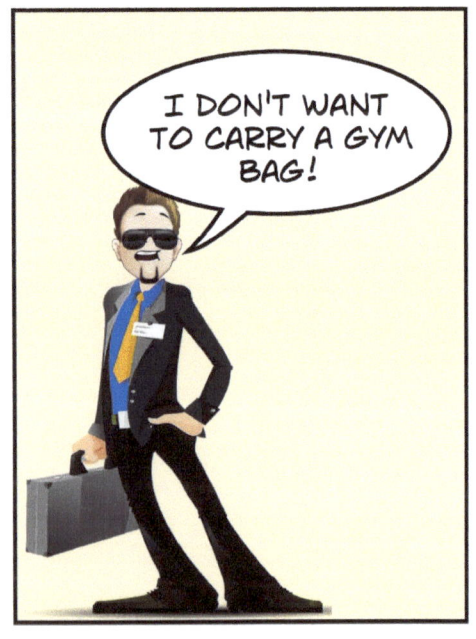

INNER FIT GIRL SAYS:

SOMETIMES GETTING THERE IS NO FUN! YOU DON'T NEED A GYM TO EXERCISE. TRY EXERCISING AT HOME OR OUTSIDE!

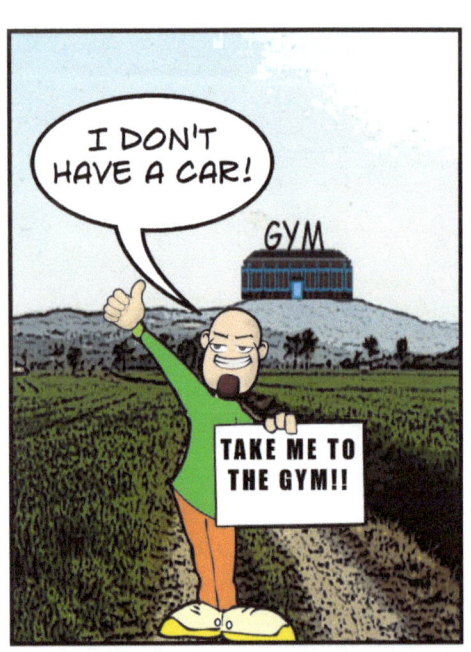

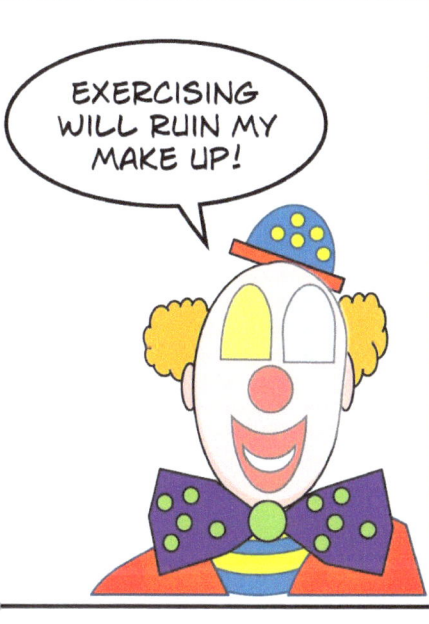

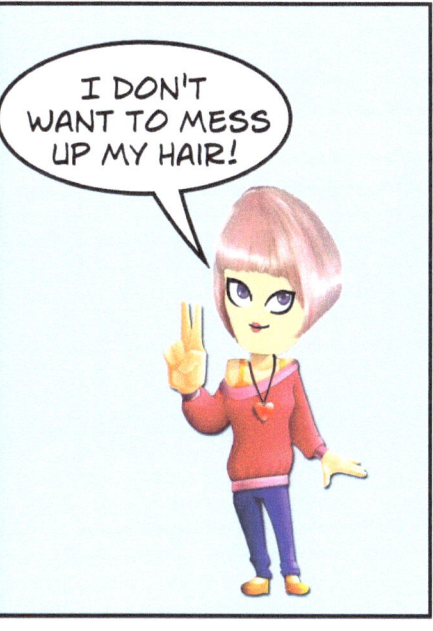

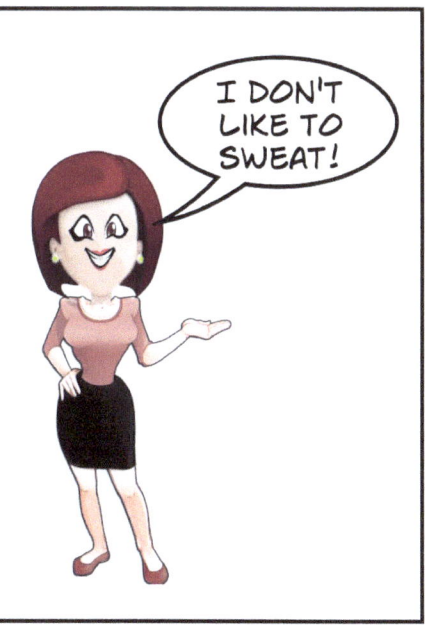

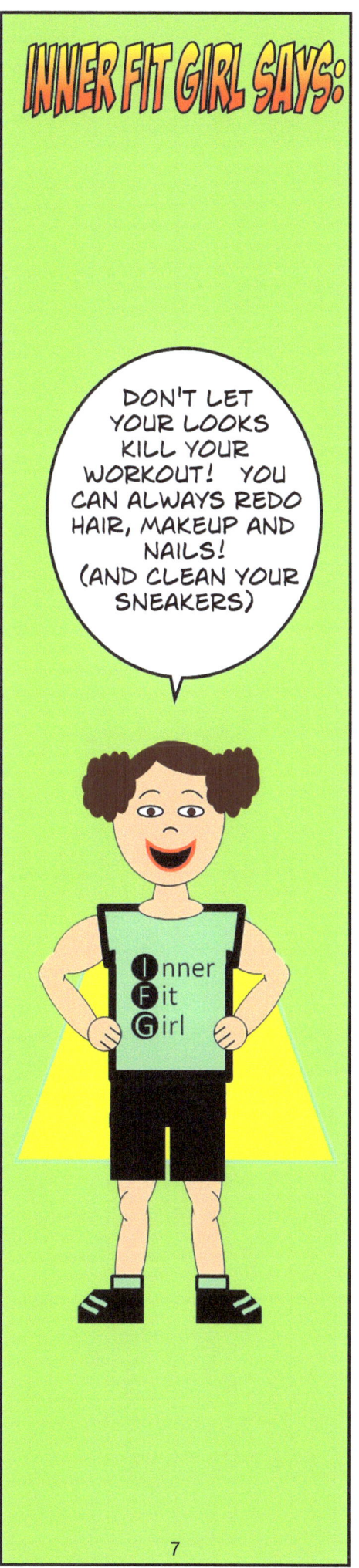

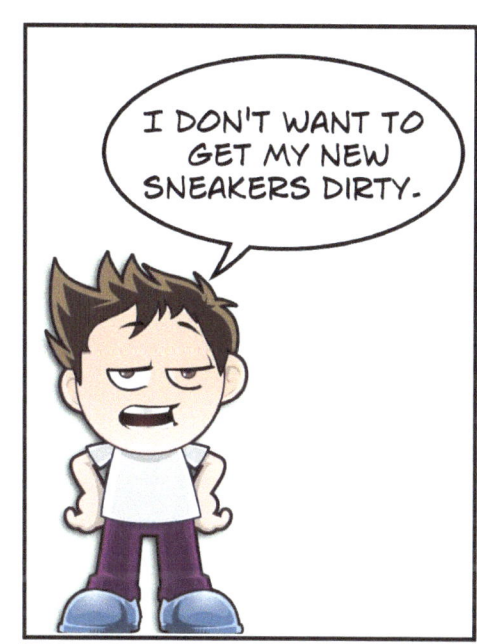

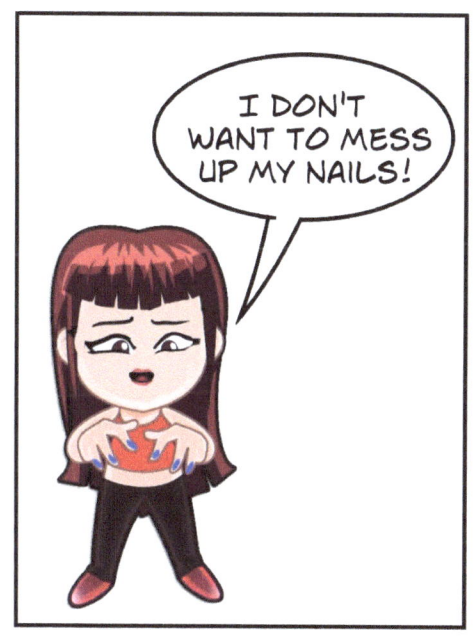

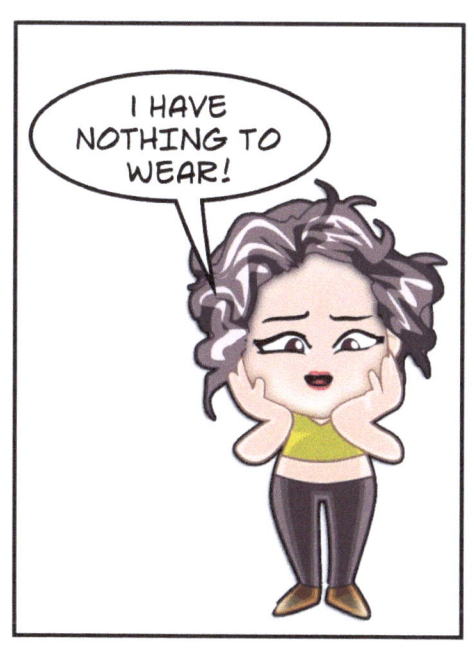

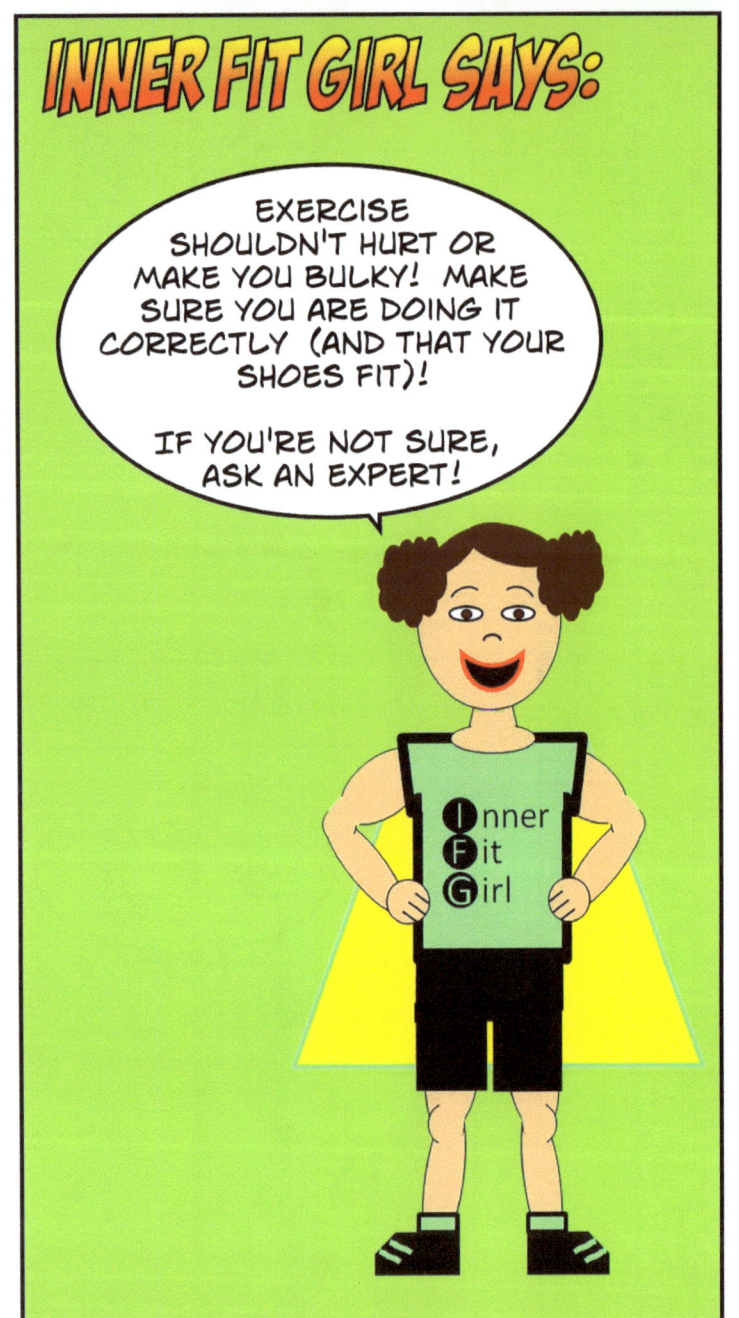

INNER FIT GIRL SAYS:

EXERCISE SHOULDN'T HURT OR MAKE YOU BULKY! MAKE SURE YOU ARE DOING IT CORRECTLY (AND THAT YOUR SHOES FIT)!

IF YOU'RE NOT SURE, ASK AN EXPERT!

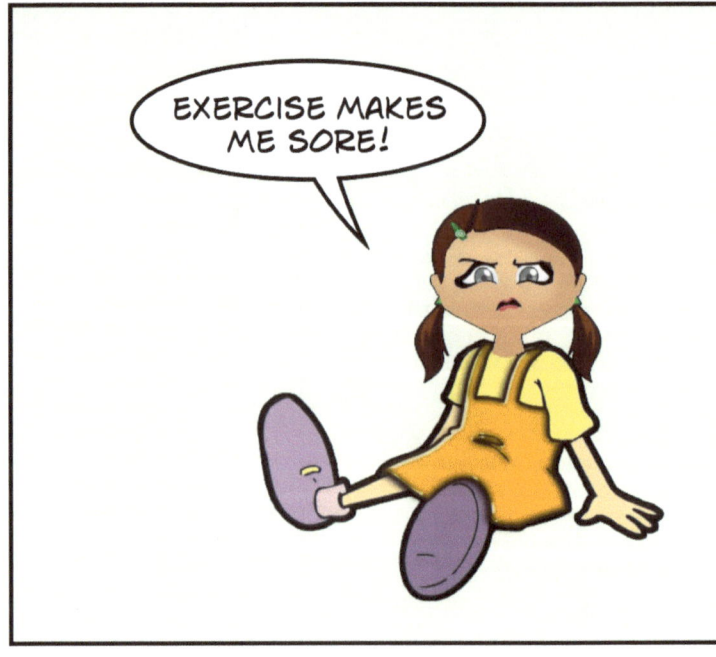

EXERCISE MAKES ME SORE!

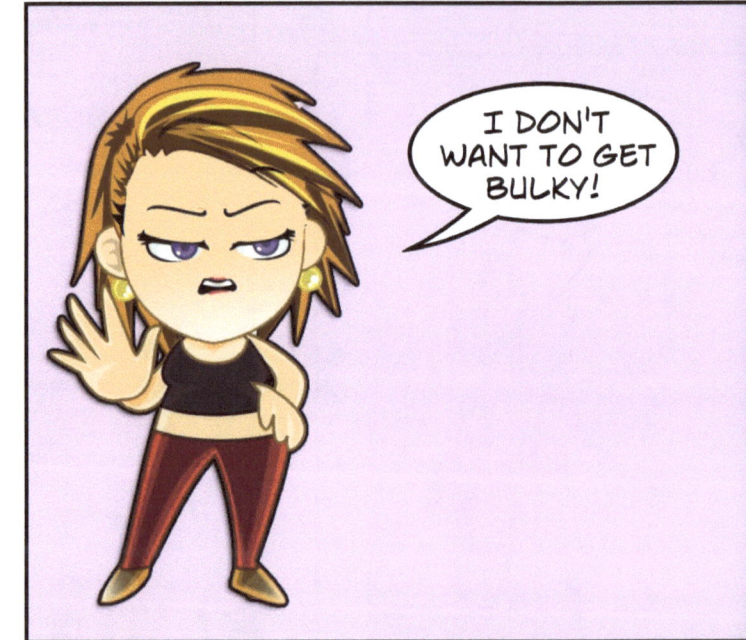

I DON'T WANT TO GET BULKY!

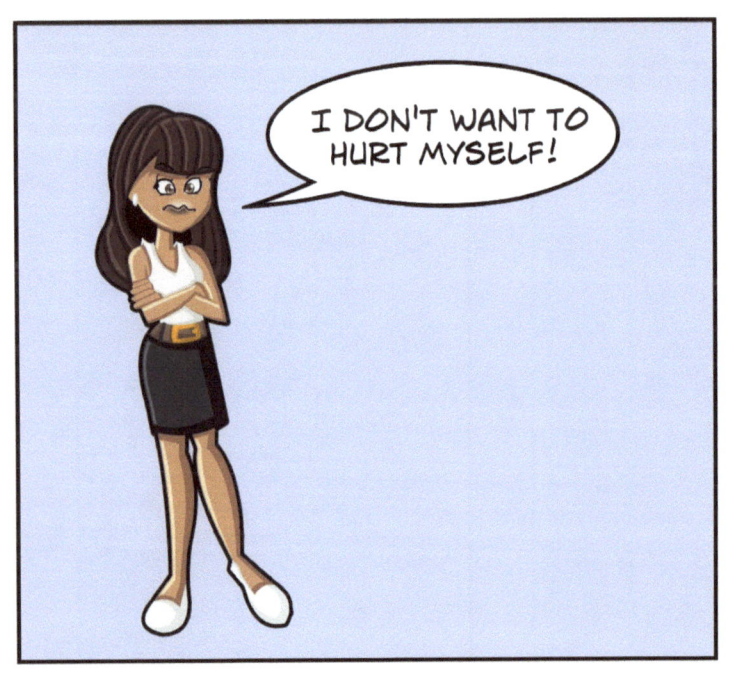

I DON'T WANT TO HURT MYSELF!

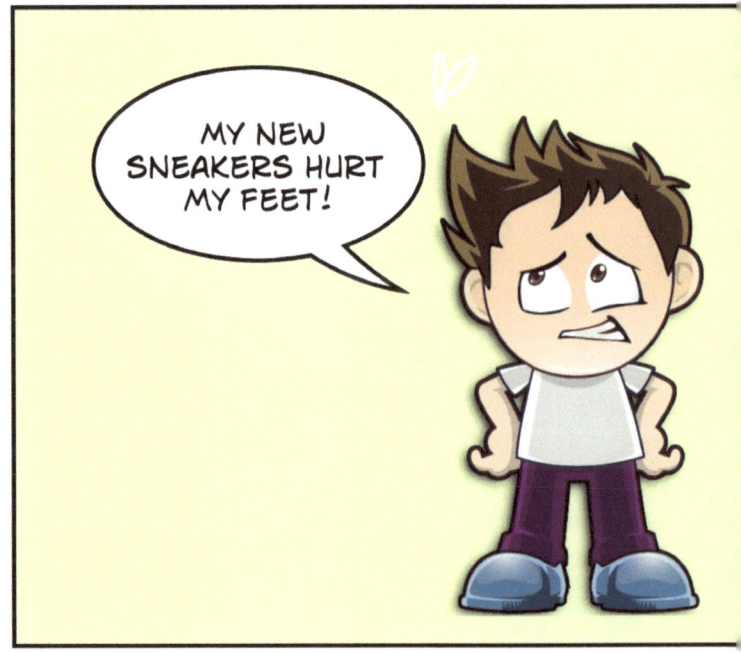

MY NEW SNEAKERS HURT MY FEET!

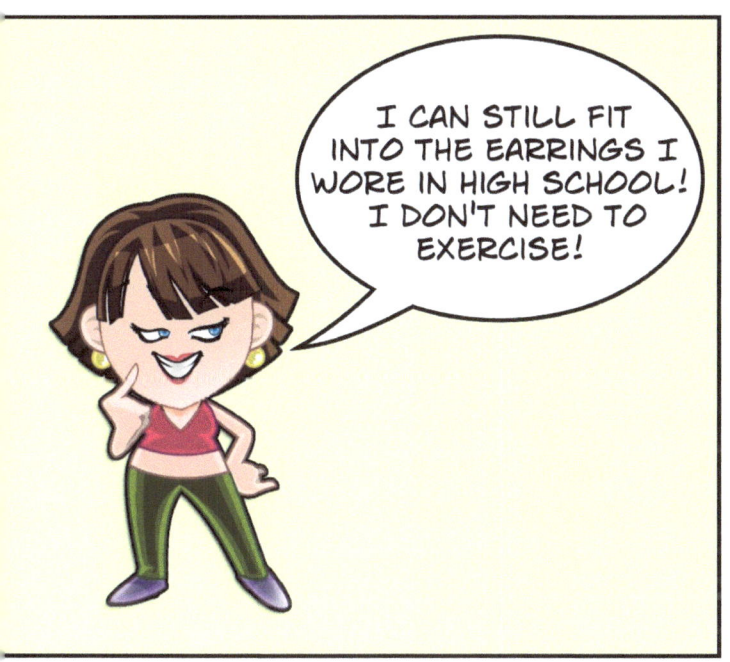

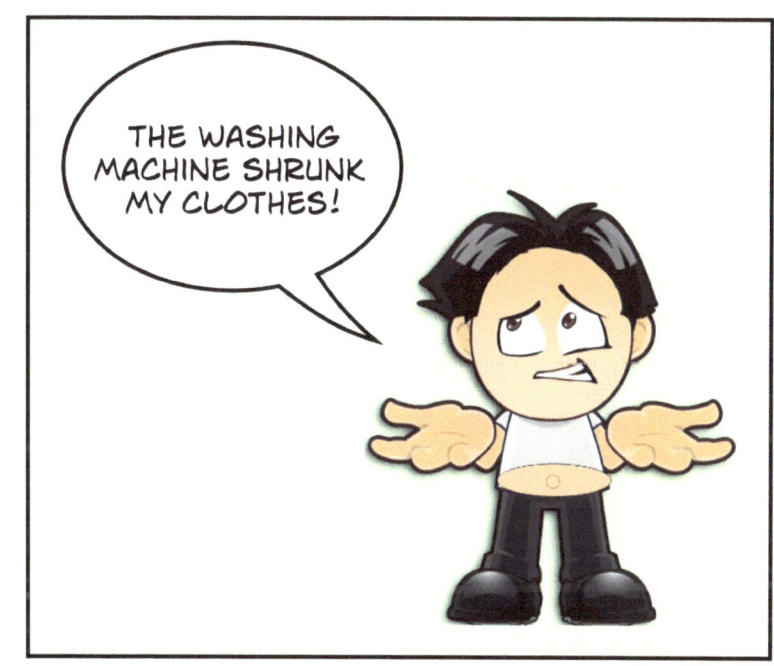

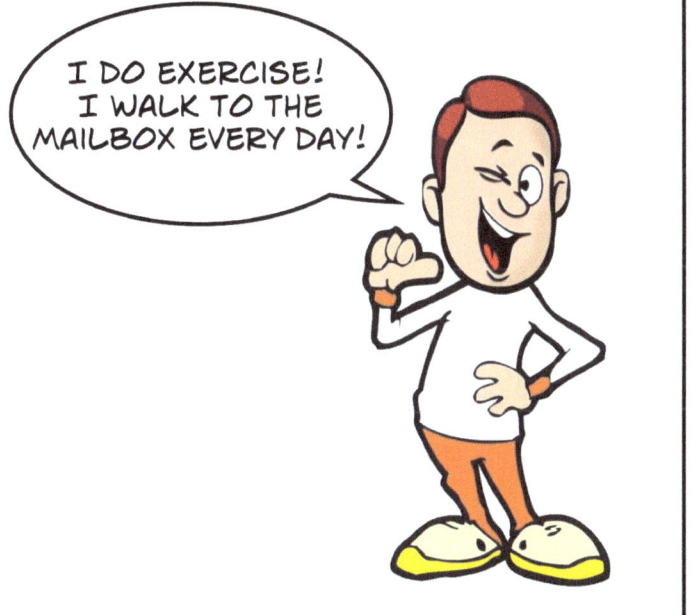

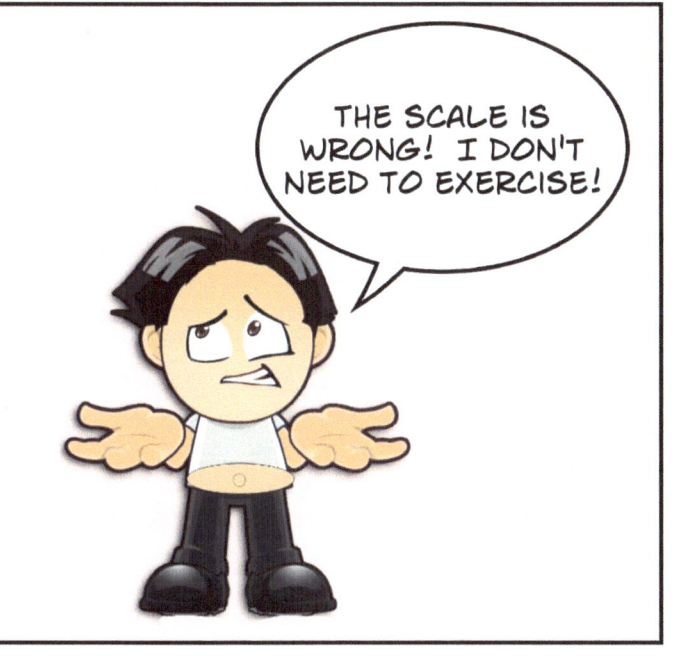

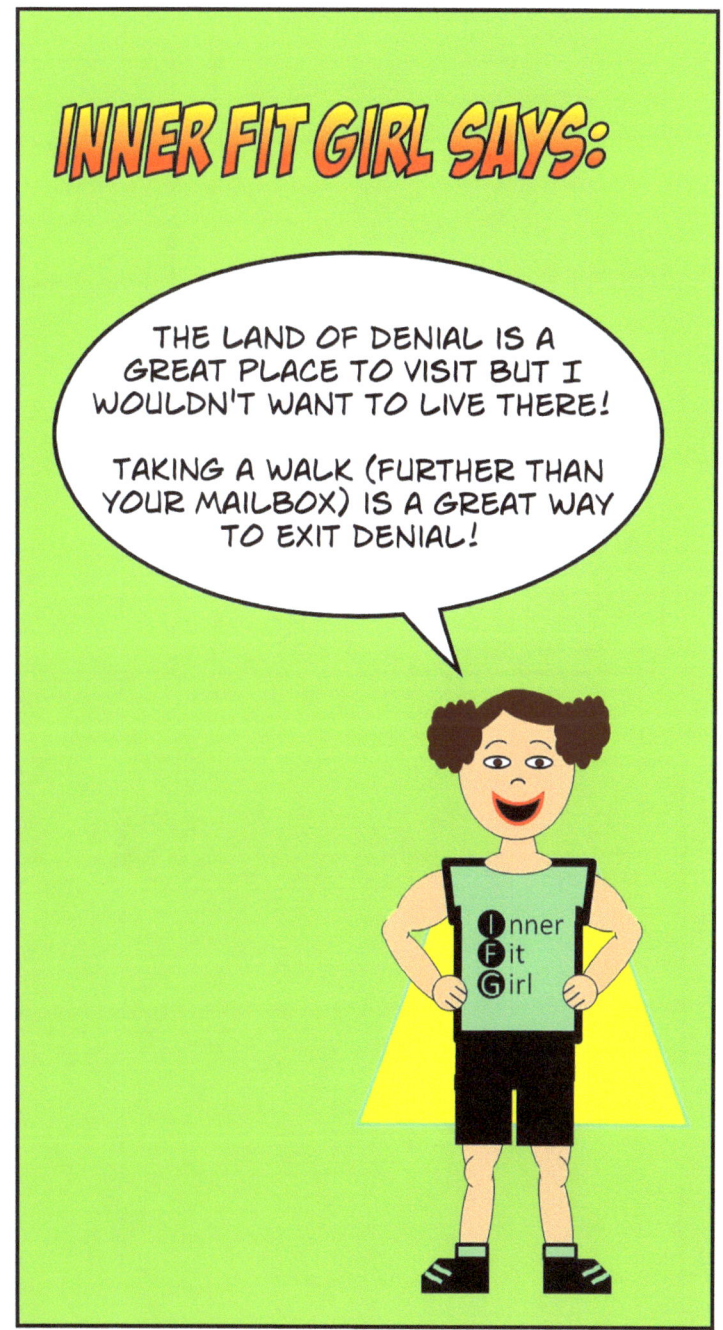

9

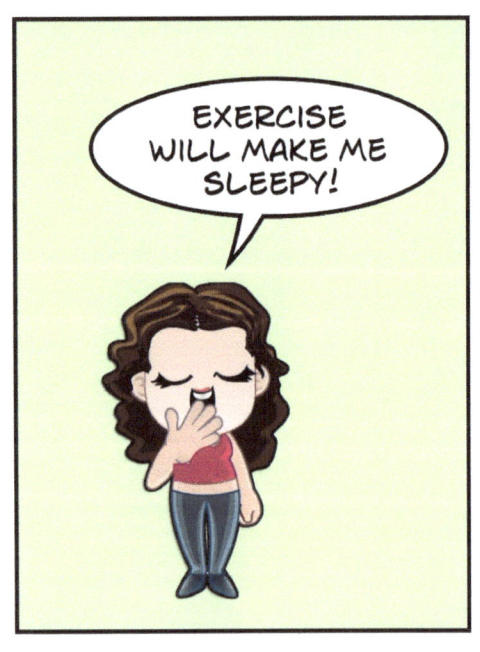

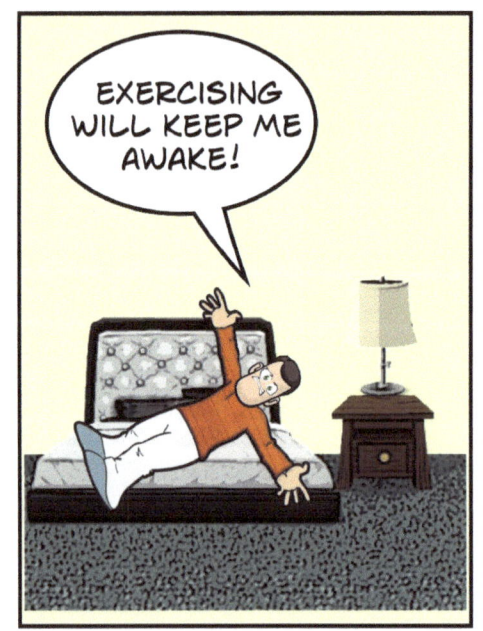

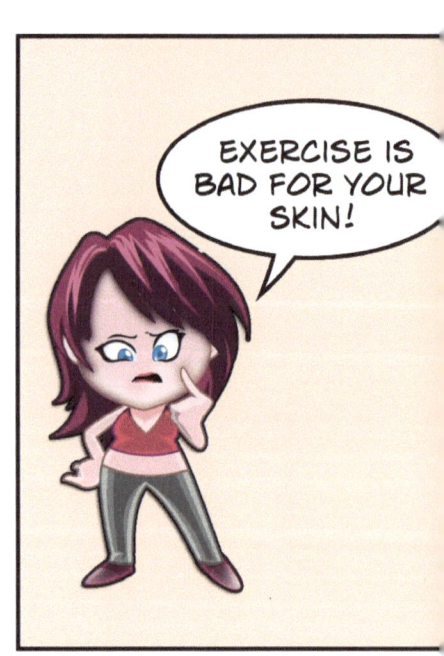

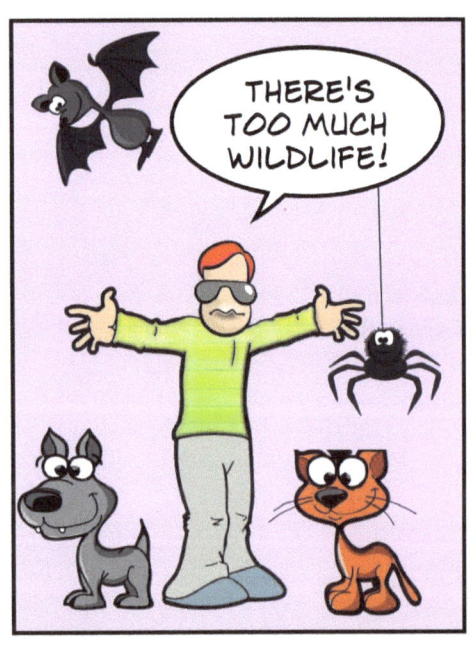

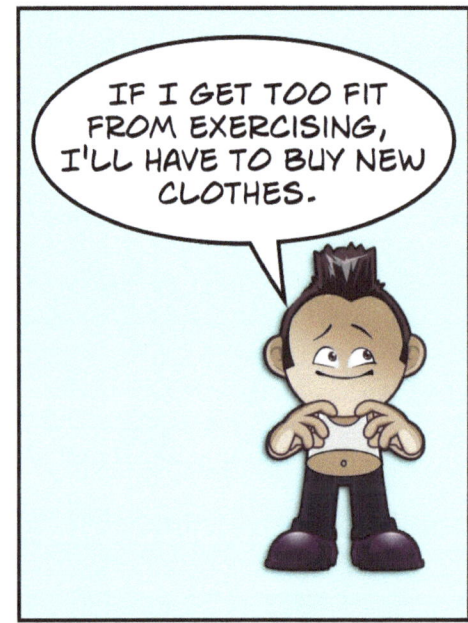

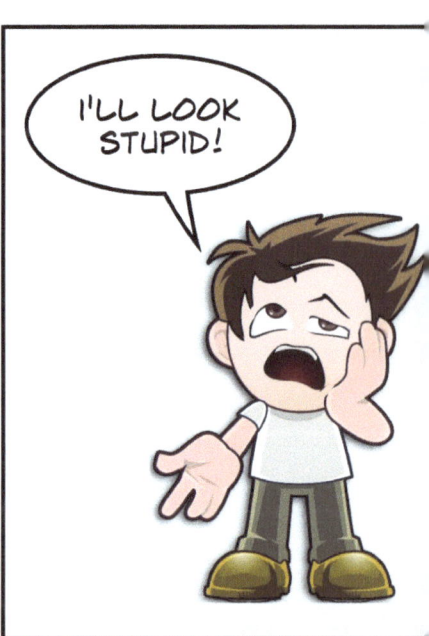

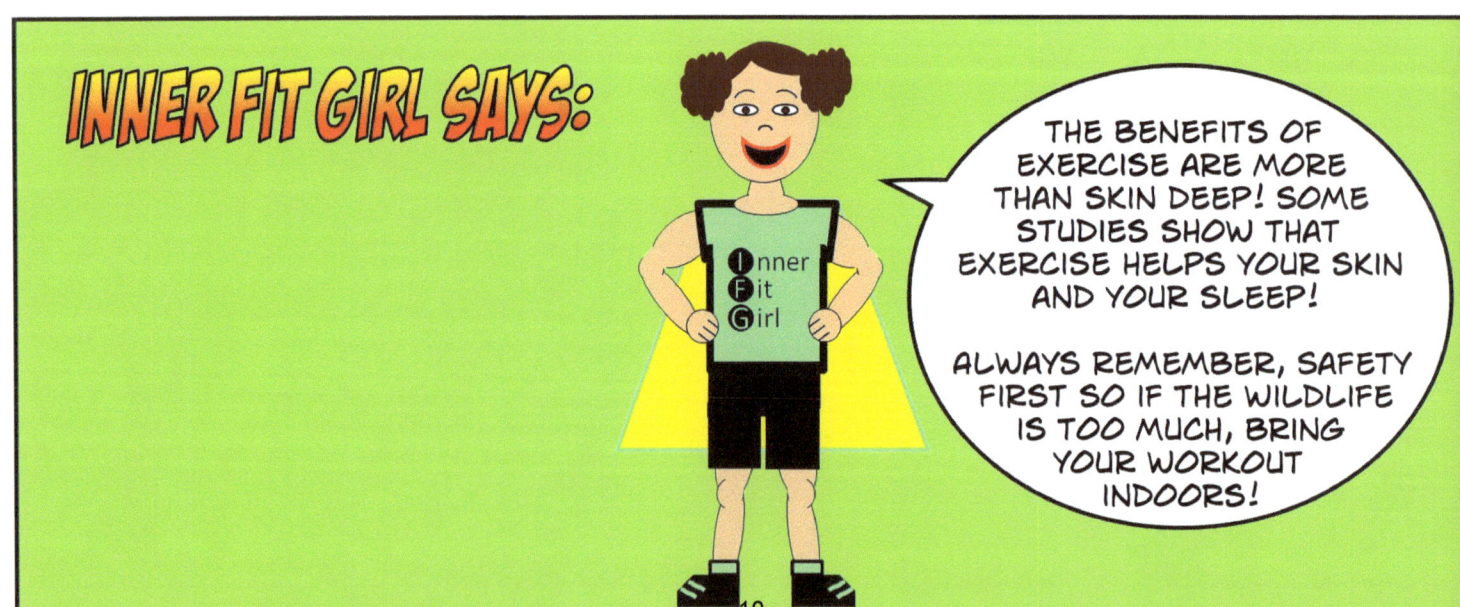

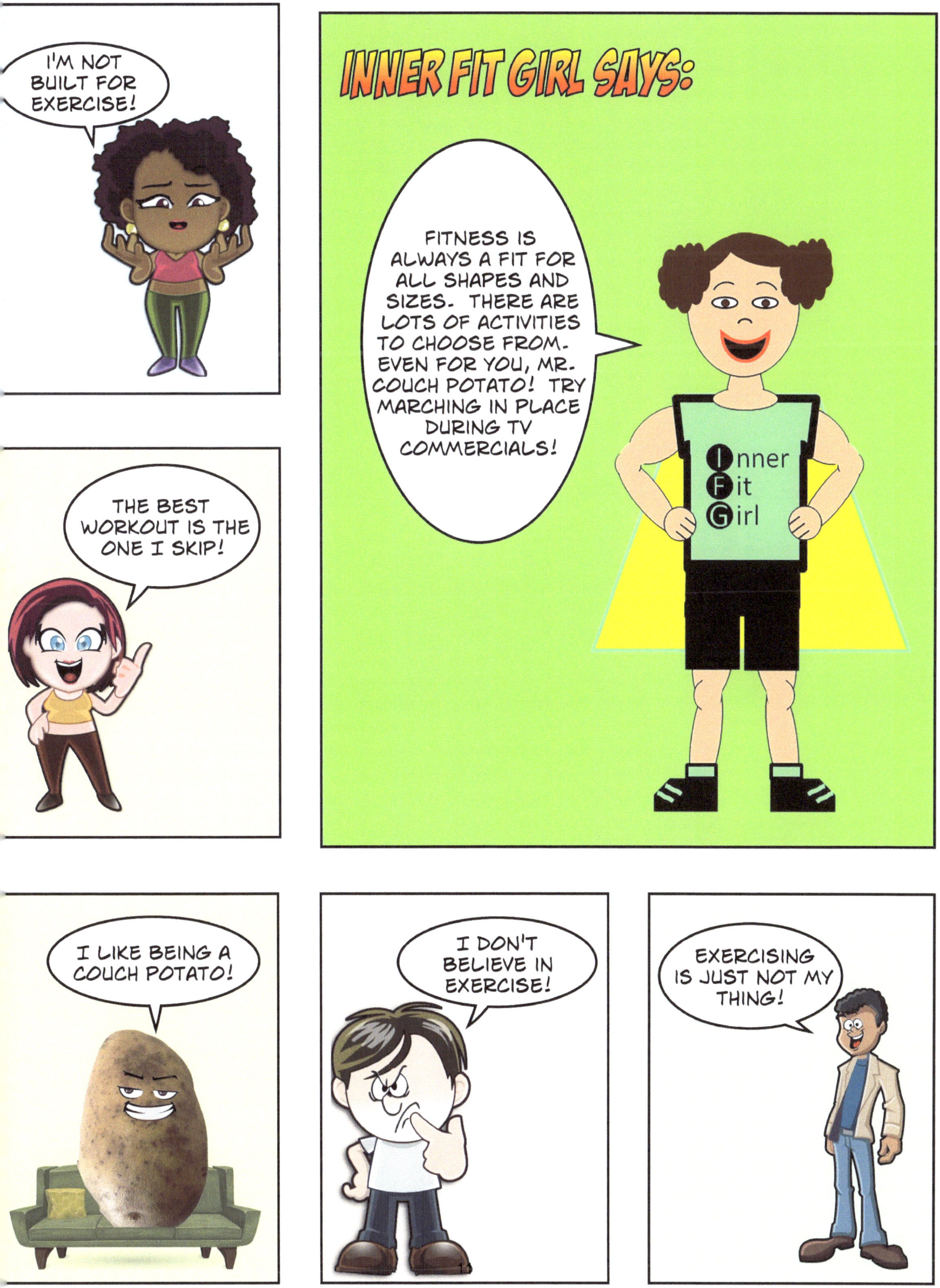

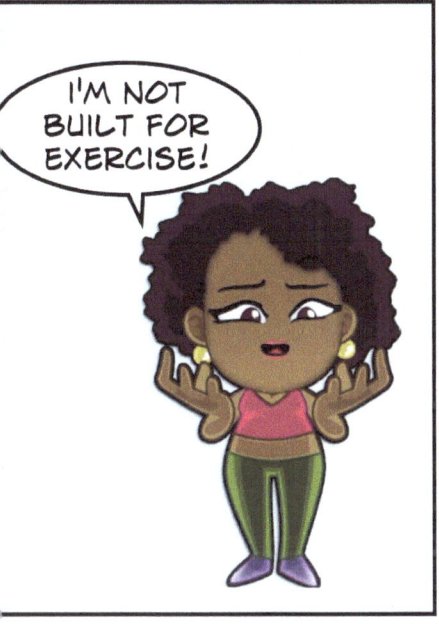

I'M NOT BUILT FOR EXERCISE!

FITNESS IS ALWAYS A FIT FOR ALL SHAPES AND SIZES. THERE ARE LOTS OF ACTIVITIES TO CHOOSE FROM. EVEN FOR YOU, MR. COUCH POTATO! TRY MARCHING IN PLACE DURING TV COMMERCIALS!

Inner Fit Girl

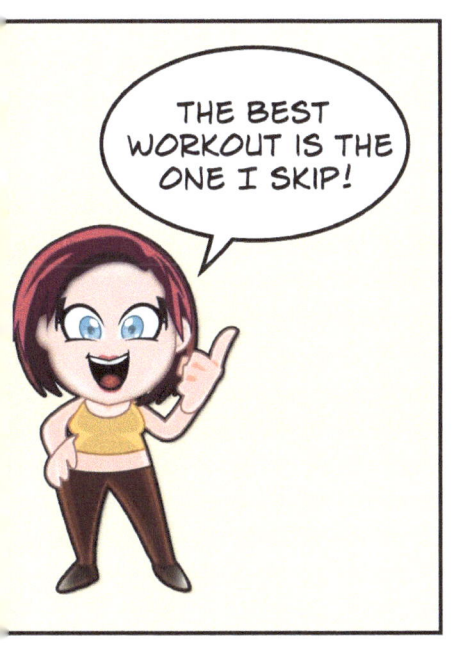

THE BEST WORKOUT IS THE ONE I SKIP!

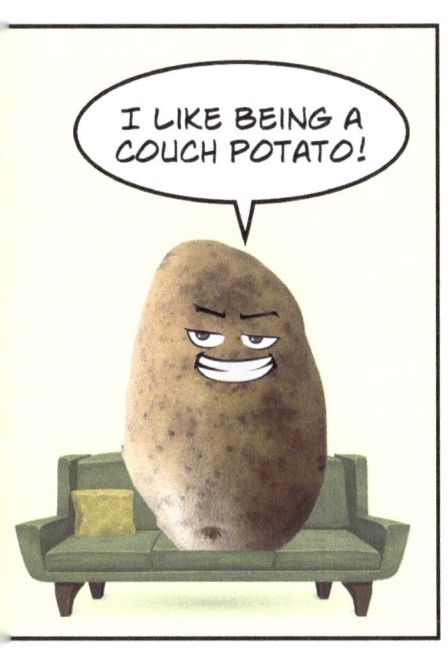

I LIKE BEING A COUCH POTATO!

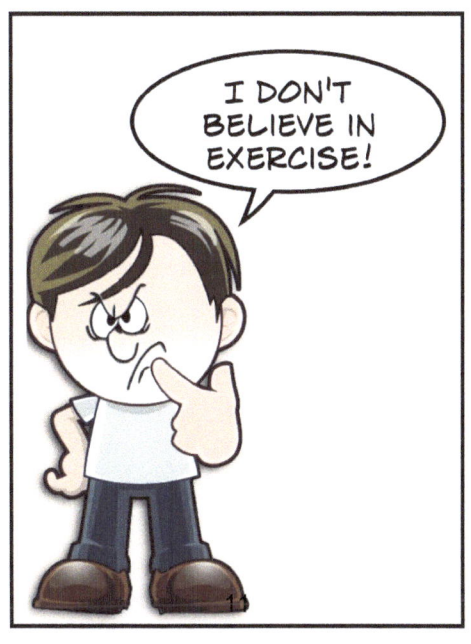

I DON'T BELIEVE IN EXERCISE!

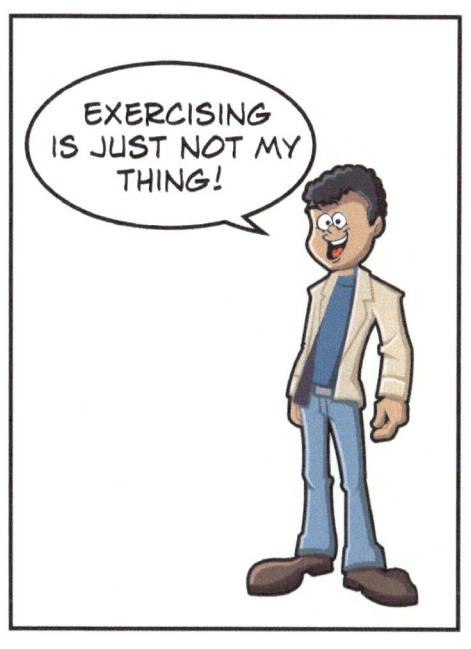

EXERCISING IS JUST NOT MY THING!

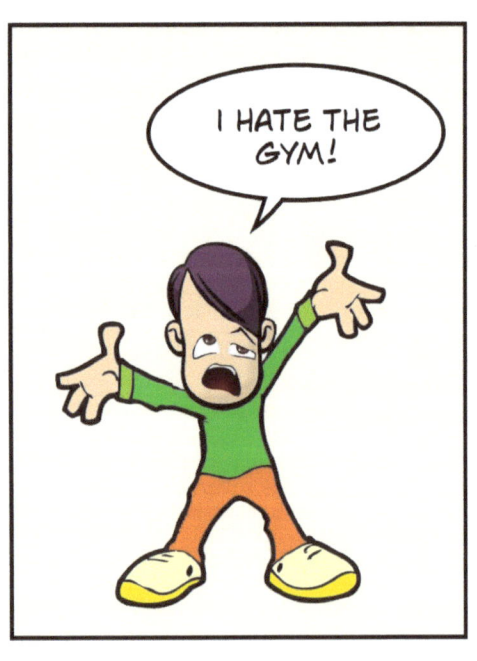

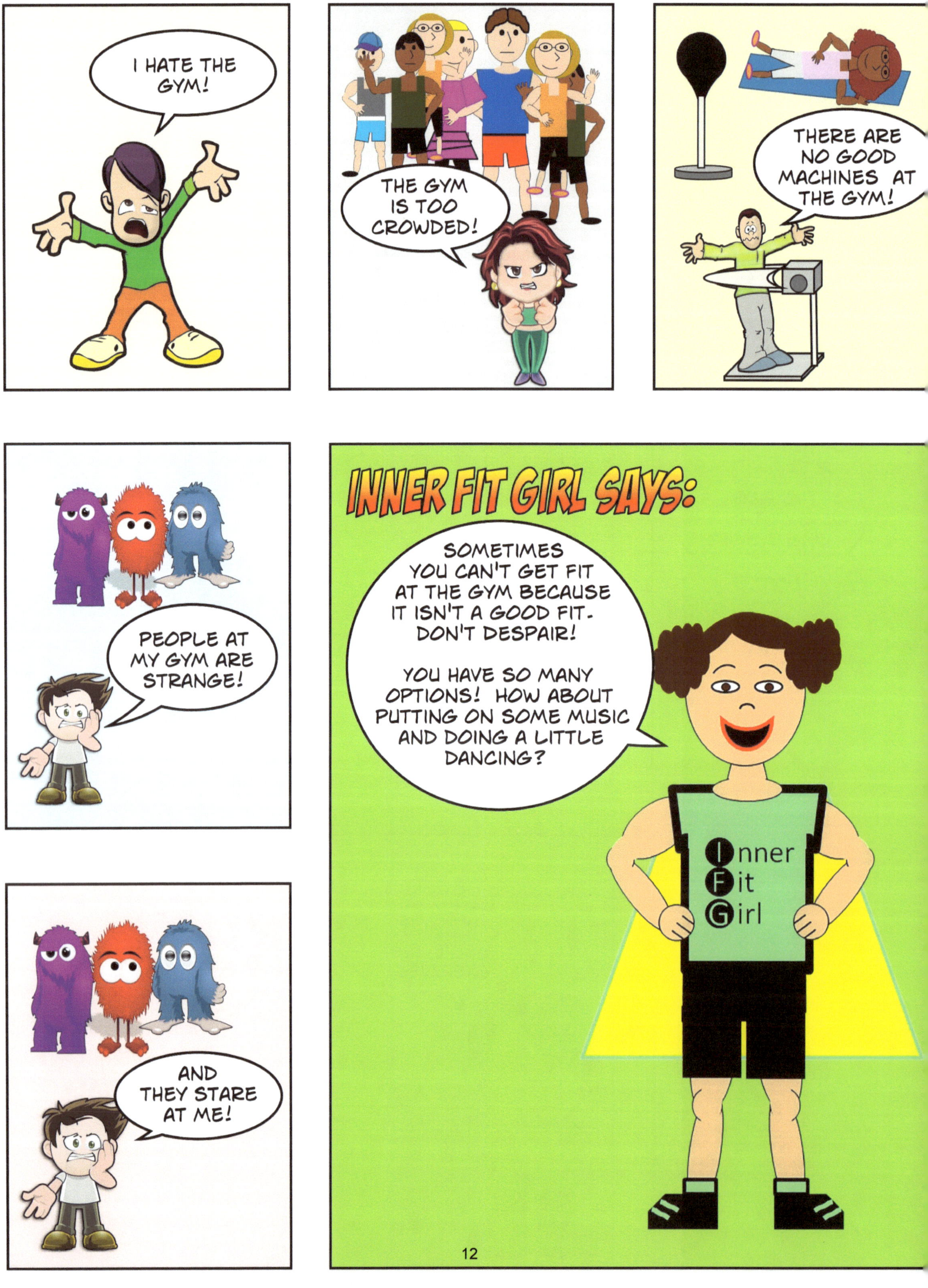

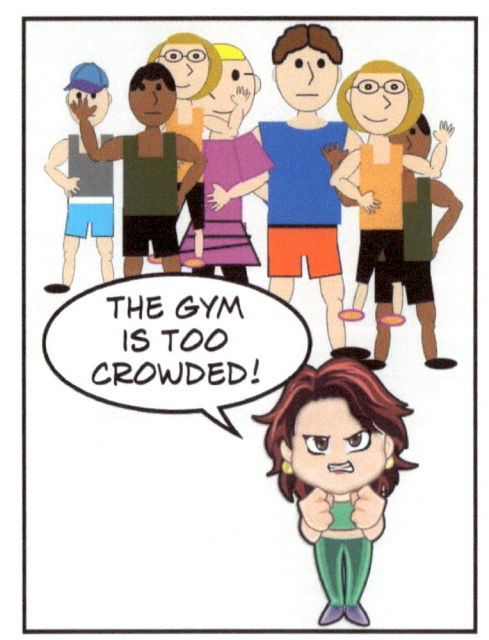

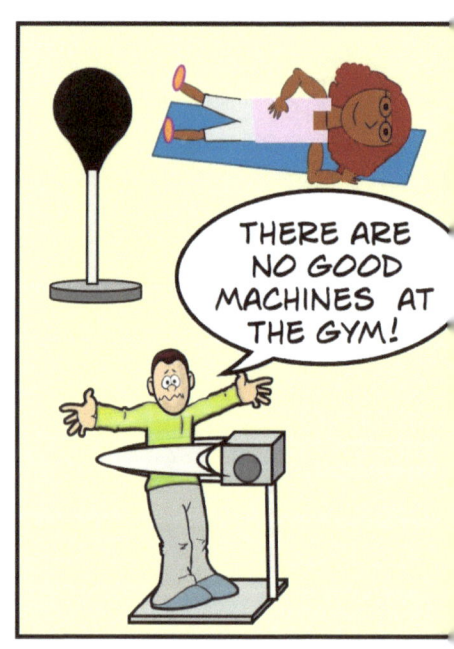

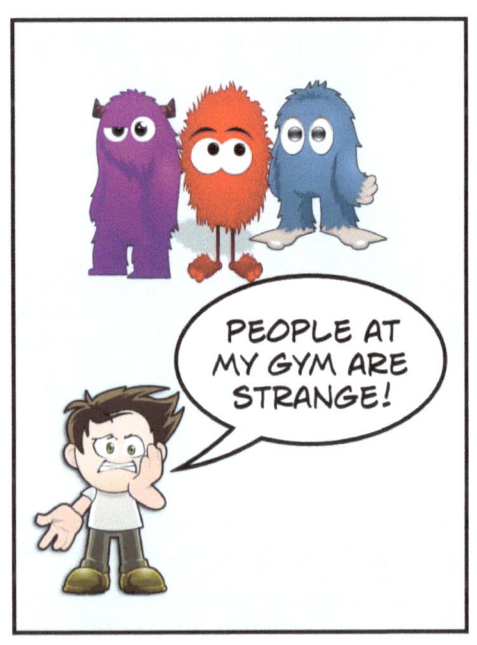

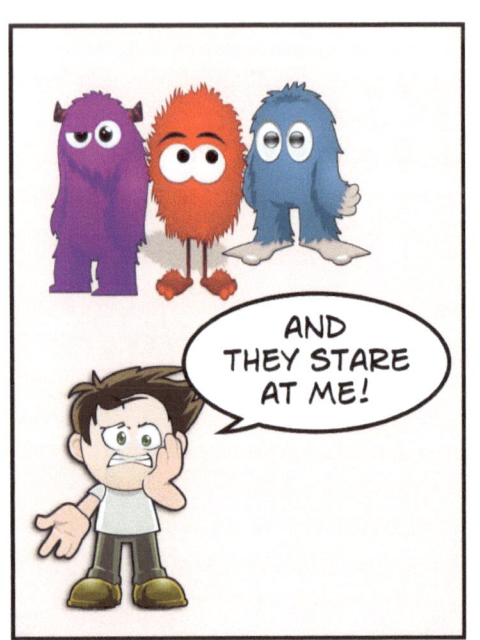

12

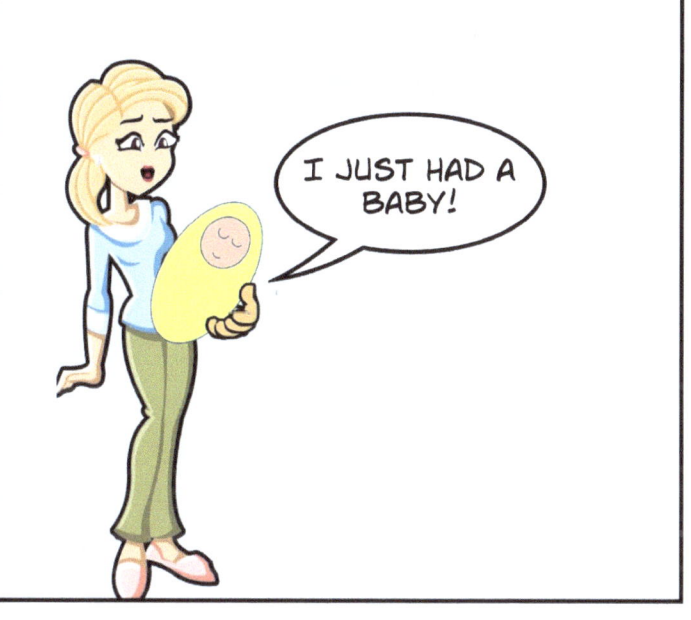

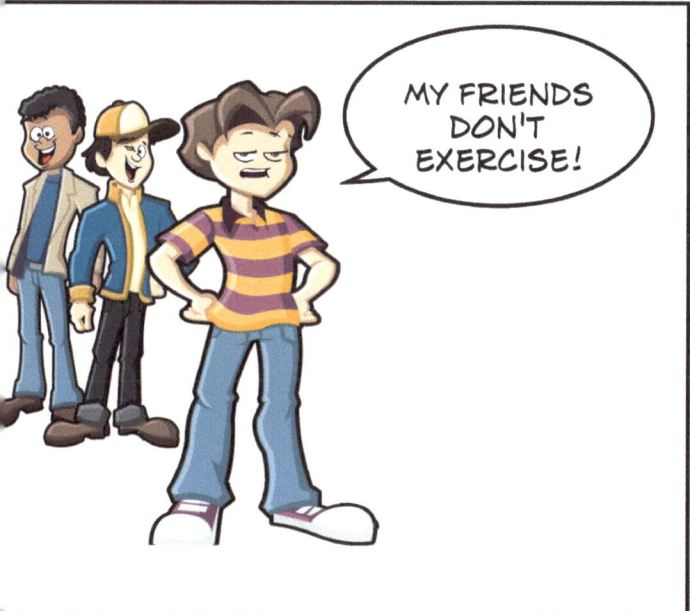

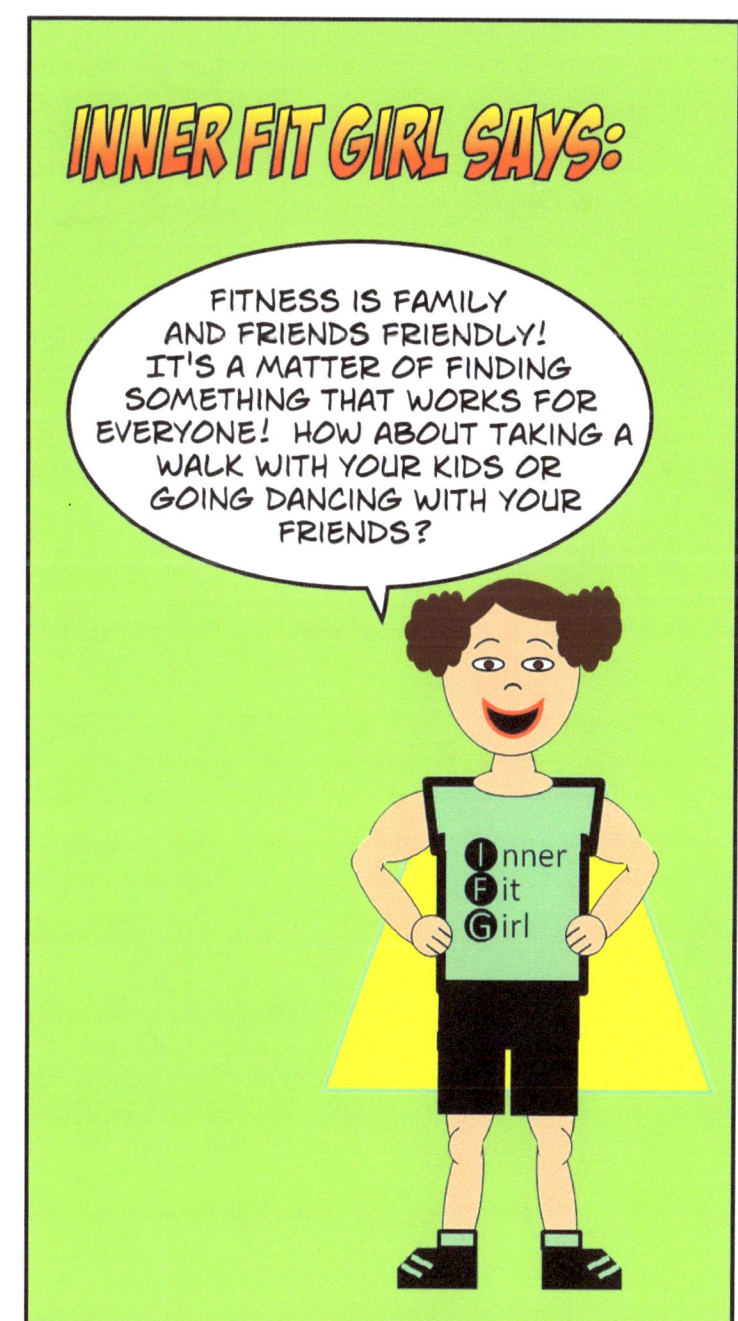

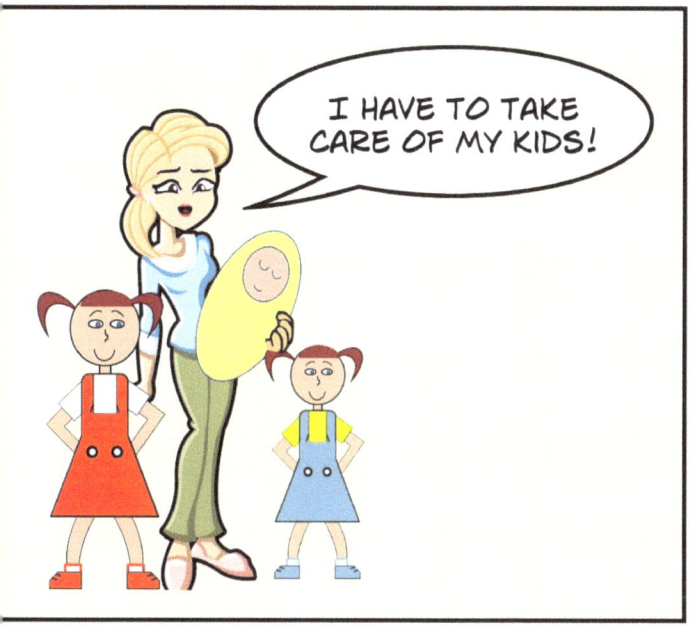

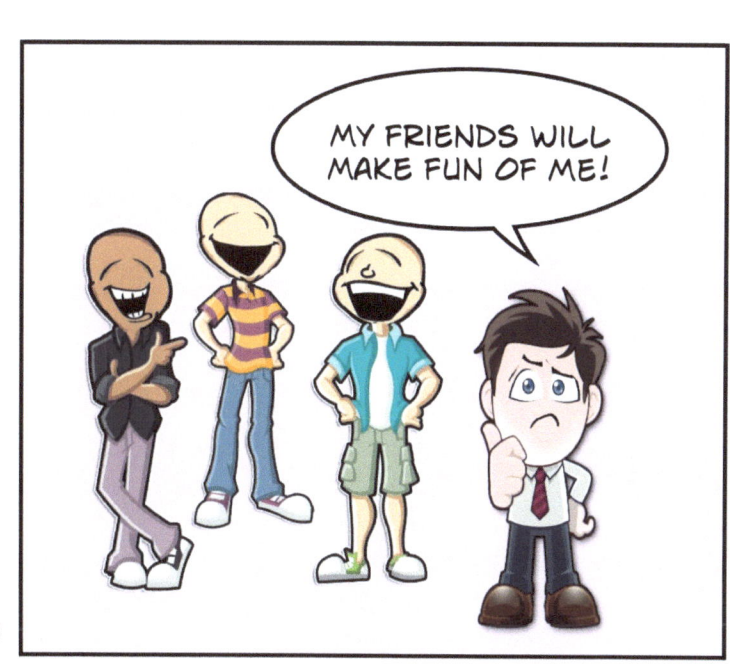

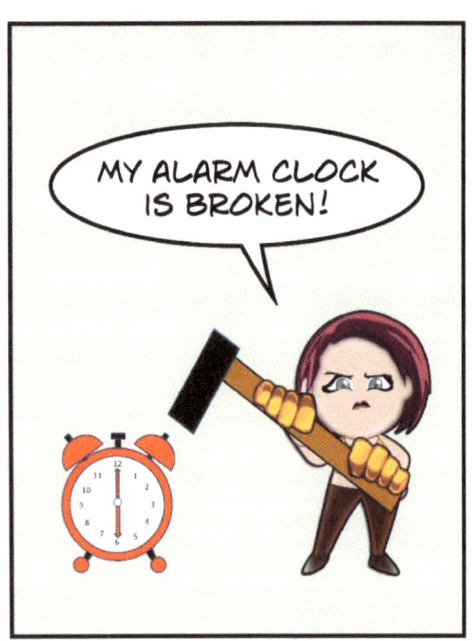

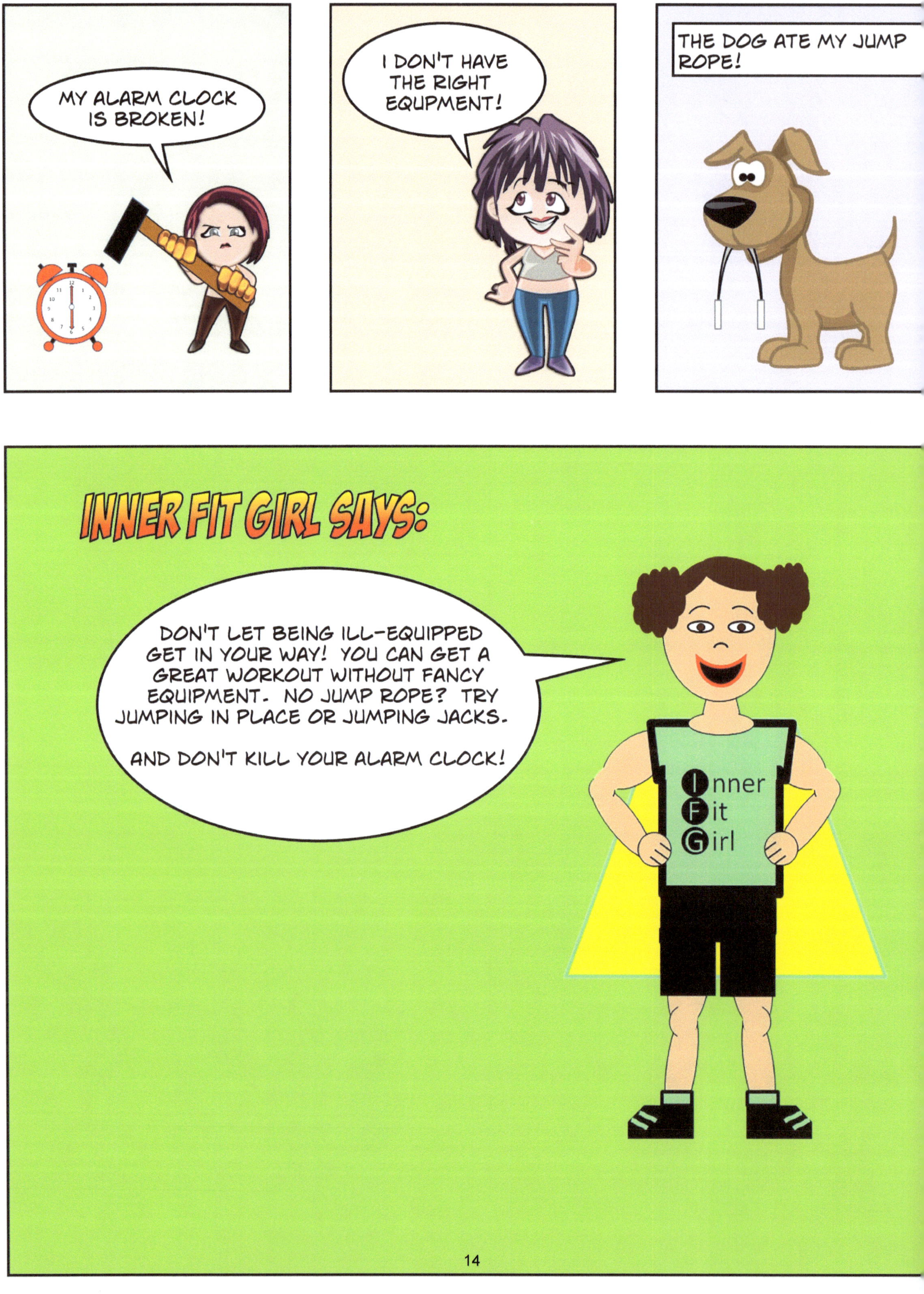

MY ALARM CLOCK IS BROKEN!

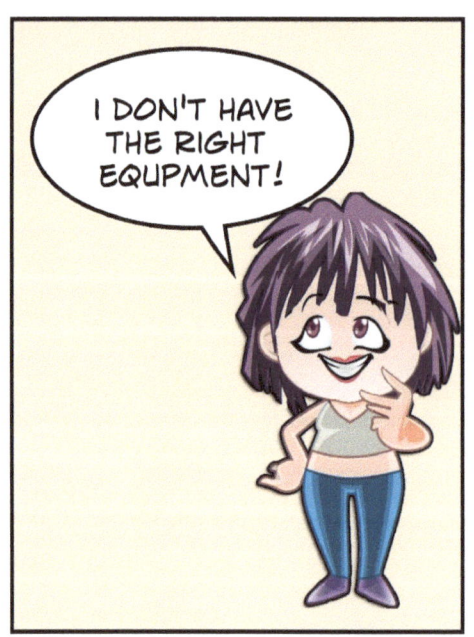

I DON'T HAVE THE RIGHT EQUPMENT!

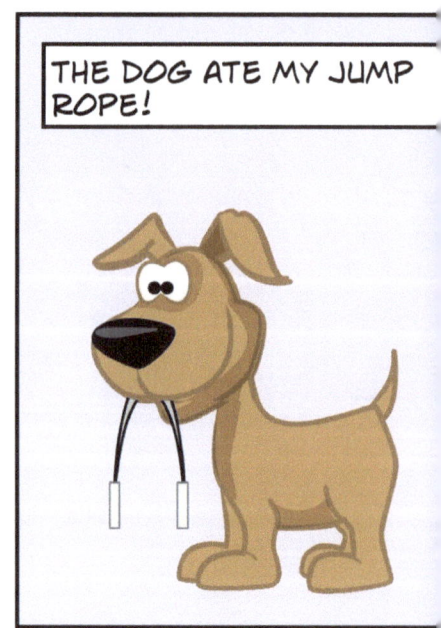

THE DOG ATE MY JUMP ROPE!

INNER FIT GIRL SAYS:

DON'T LET BEING ILL—EQUIPPED GET IN YOUR WAY! YOU CAN GET A GREAT WORKOUT WITHOUT FANCY EQUIPMENT. NO JUMP ROPE? TRY JUMPING IN PLACE OR JUMPING JACKS.

AND DON'T KILL YOUR ALARM CLOCK!

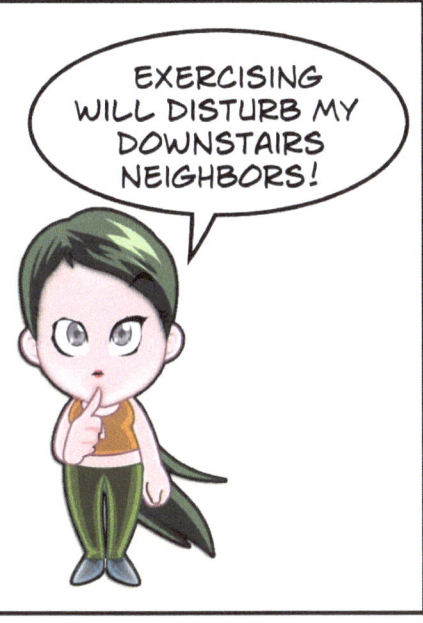

EXERCISING WILL DISTURB MY DOWNSTAIRS NEIGHBORS!

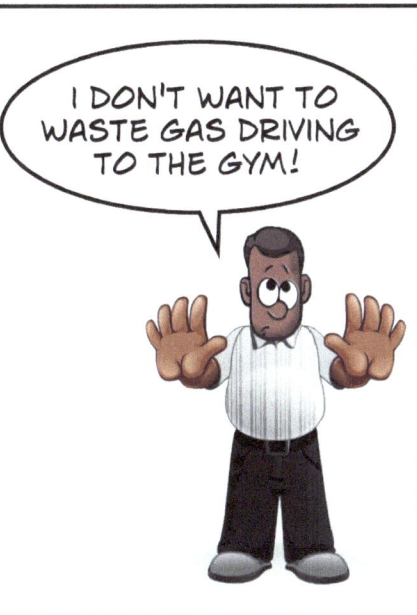

I DON'T WANT TO WASTE GAS DRIVING TO THE GYM!

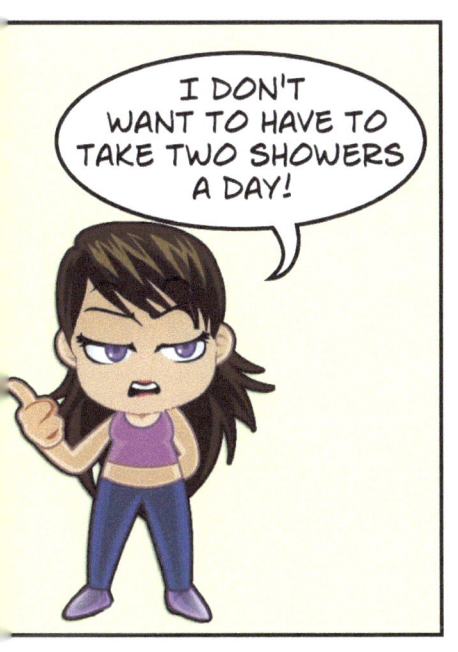

I DON'T WANT TO HAVE TO TAKE TWO SHOWERS A DAY!

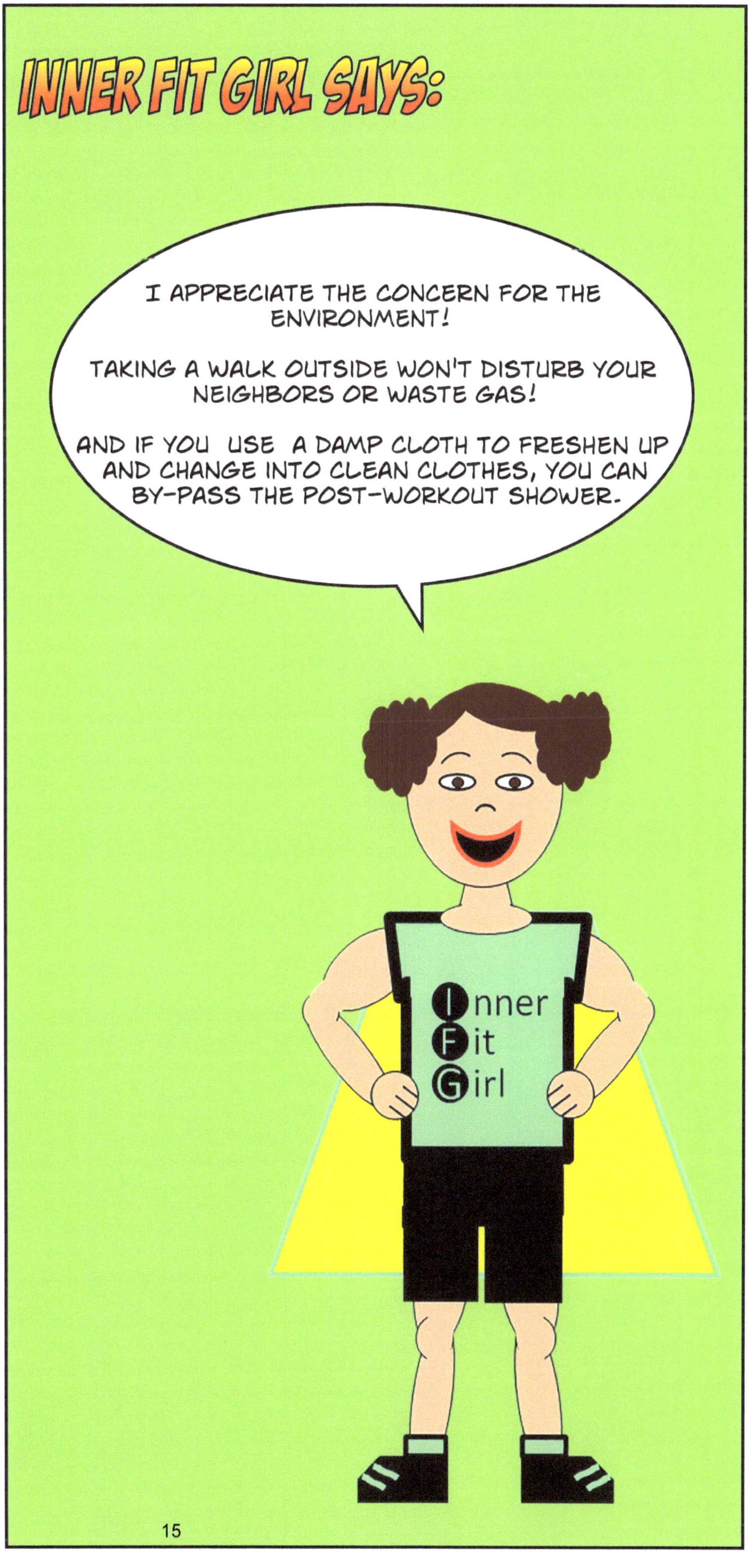

INNER FIT GIRL SAYS:

I APPRECIATE THE CONCERN FOR THE ENVIRONMENT!

TAKING A WALK OUTSIDE WON'T DISTURB YOUR NEIGHBORS OR WASTE GAS!

AND IF YOU USE A DAMP CLOTH TO FRESHEN UP AND CHANGE INTO CLEAN CLOTHES, YOU CAN BY-PASS THE POST-WORKOUT SHOWER.

Inner Fit Girl

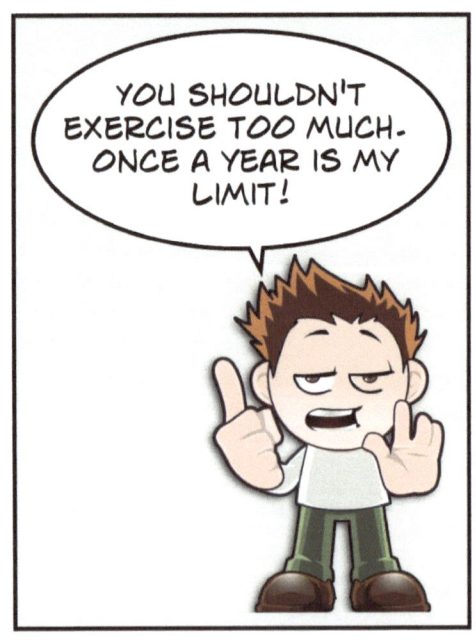

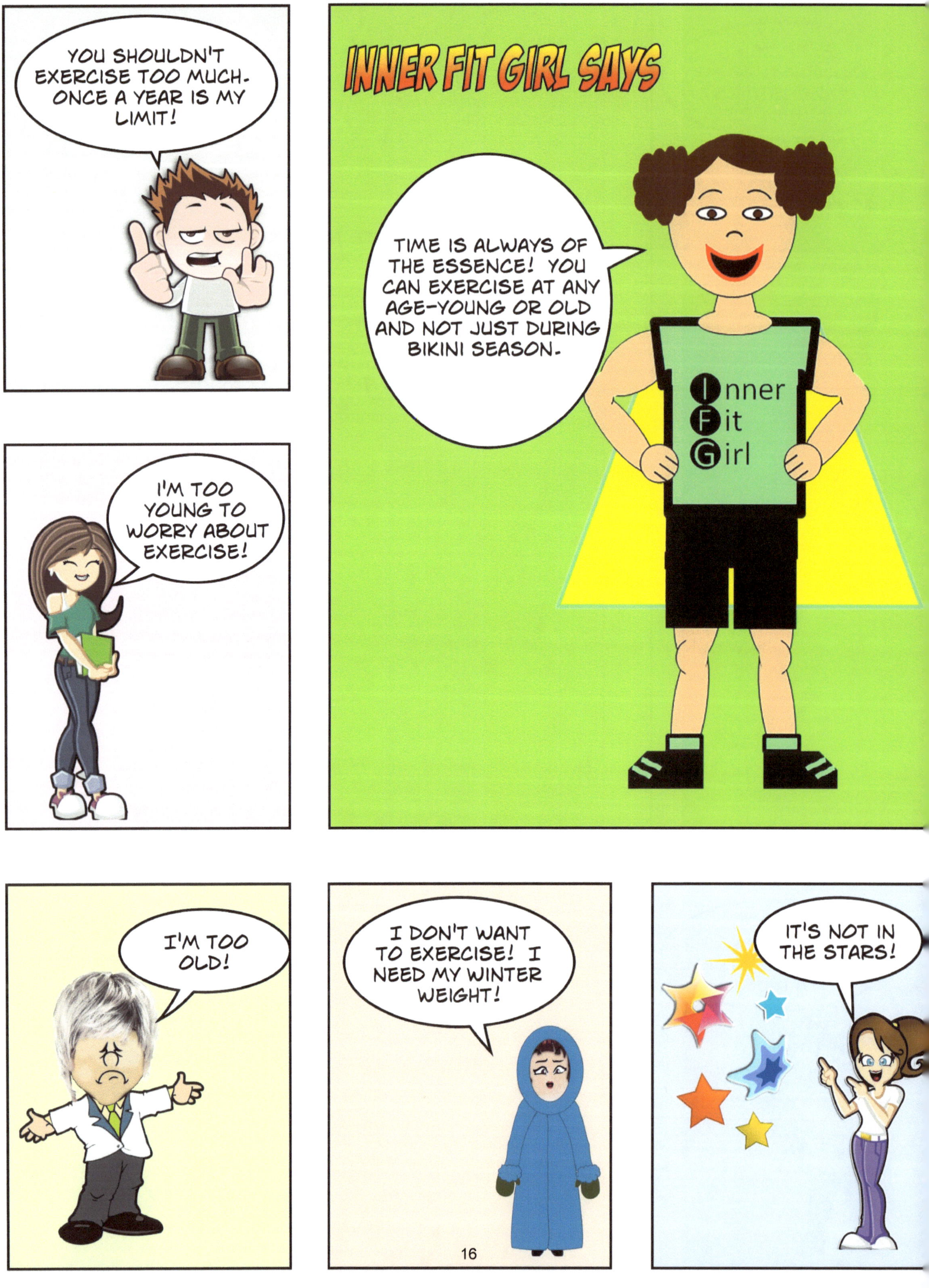

YOU SHOULDN'T EXERCISE TOO MUCH. ONCE A YEAR IS MY LIMIT!

INNER FIT GIRL SAYS

TIME IS ALWAYS OF THE ESSENCE! YOU CAN EXERCISE AT ANY AGE–YOUNG OR OLD AND NOT JUST DURING BIKINI SEASON.

Inner
Fit
Girl

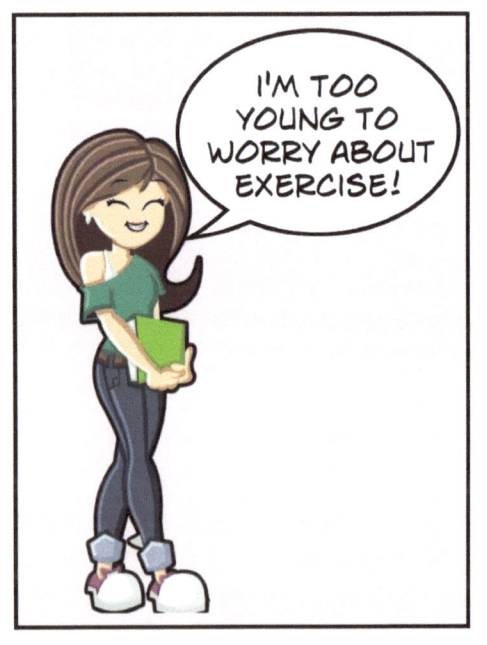

I'M TOO YOUNG TO WORRY ABOUT EXERCISE!

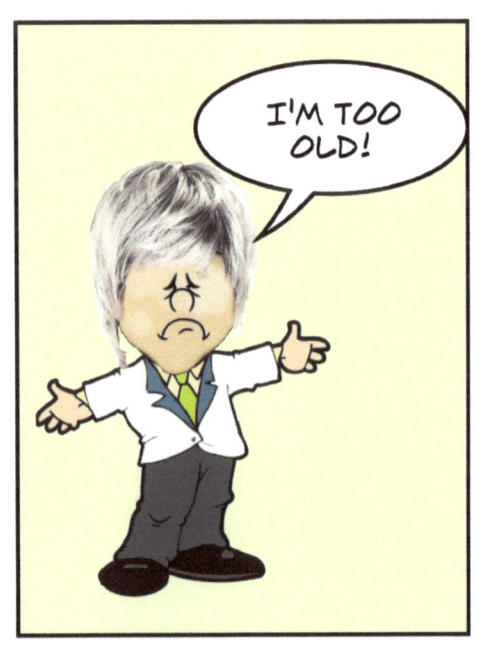

I'M TOO OLD!

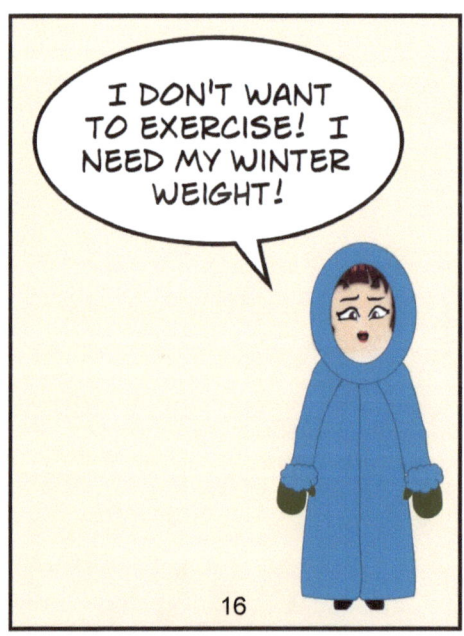

I DON'T WANT TO EXERCISE! I NEED MY WINTER WEIGHT!

16

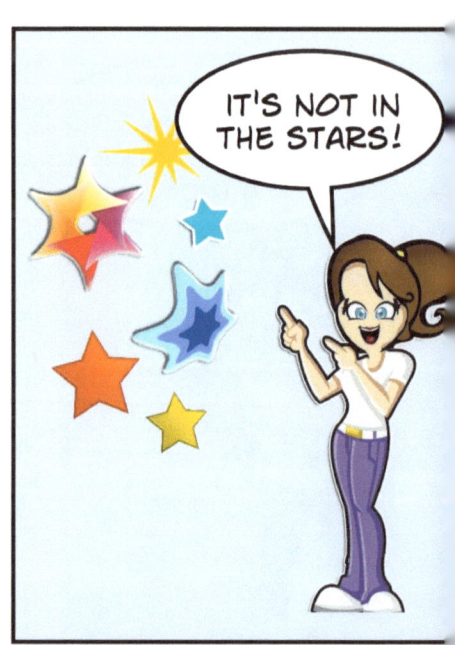

IT'S NOT IN THE STARS!

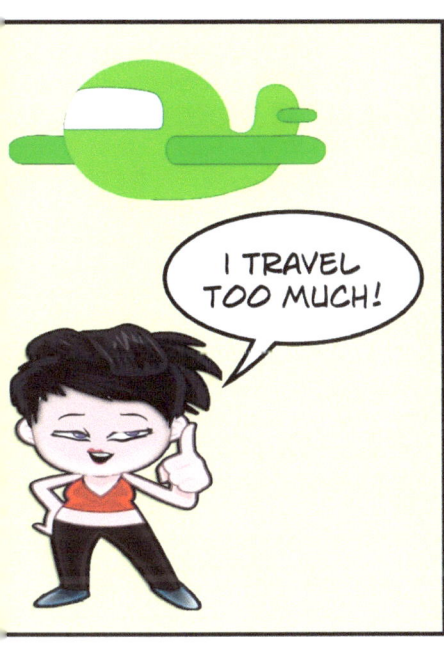

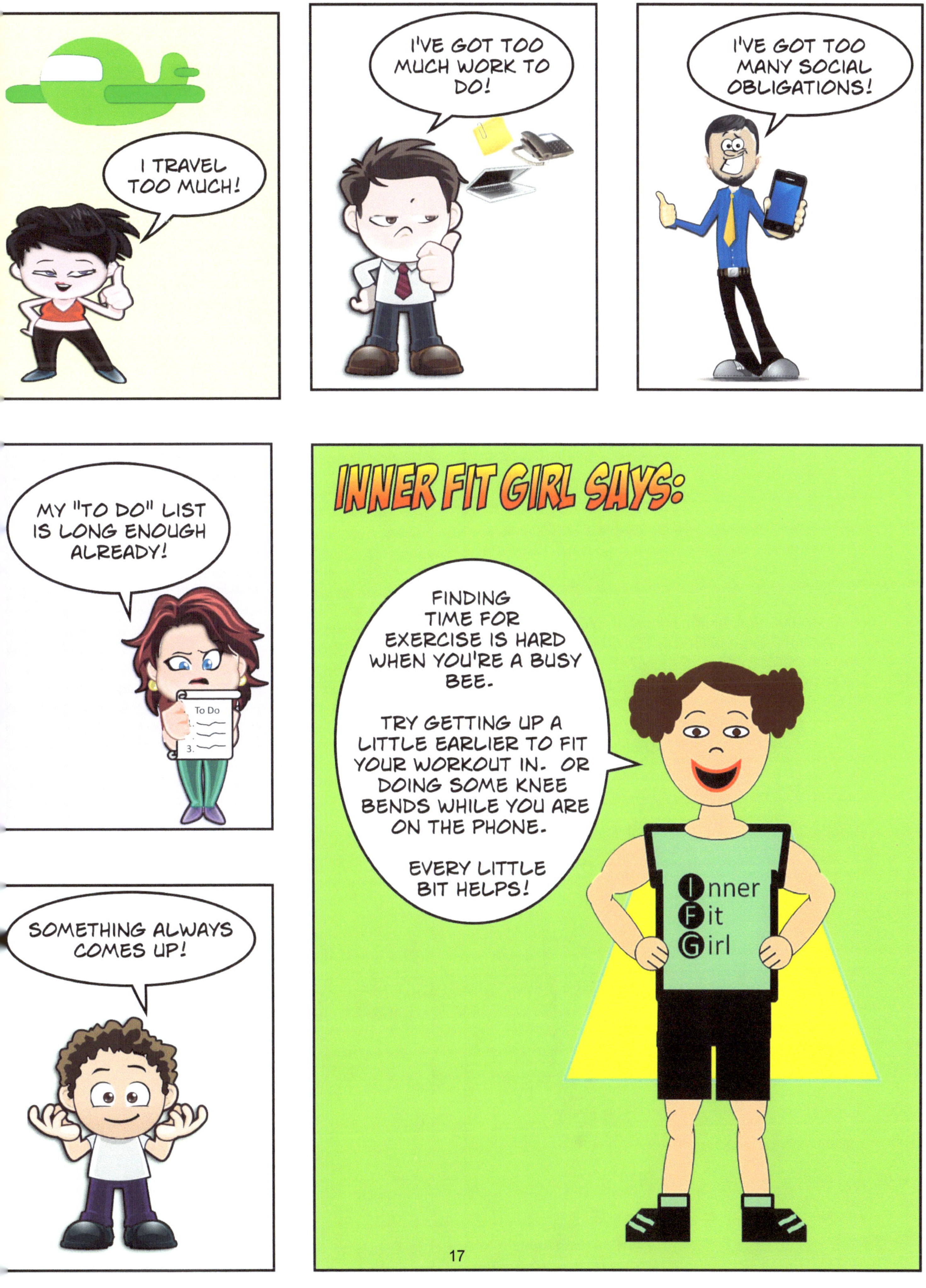

I TRAVEL TOO MUCH!

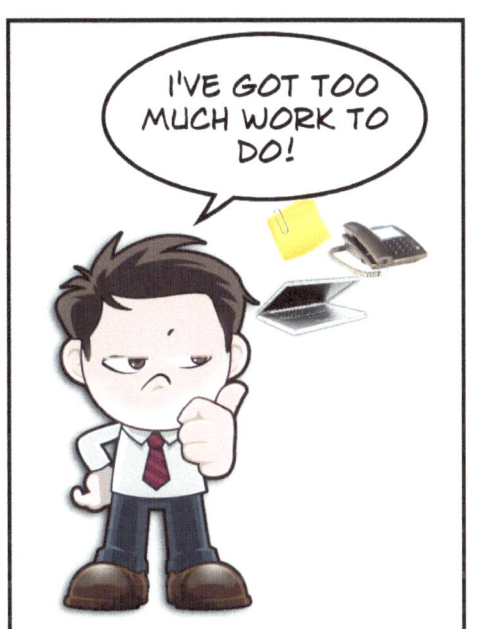

I'VE GOT TOO MUCH WORK TO DO!

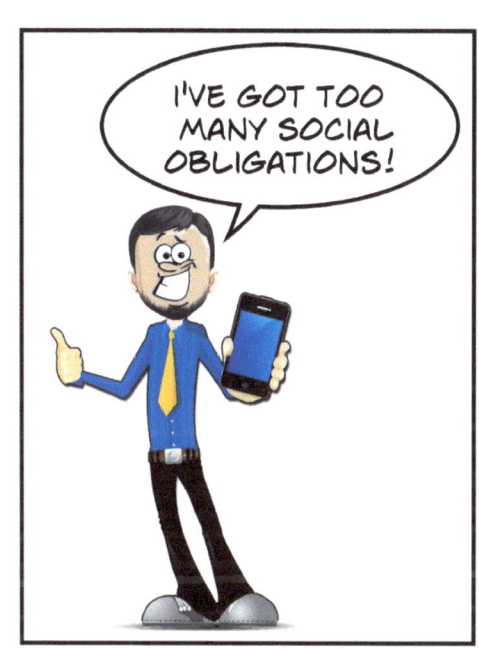

I'VE GOT TOO MANY SOCIAL OBLIGATIONS!

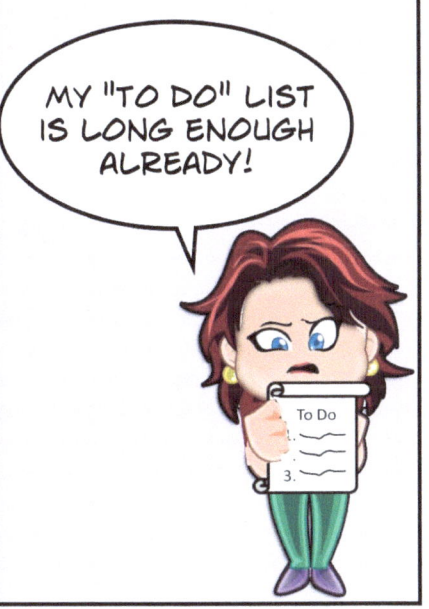

MY "TO DO" LIST IS LONG ENOUGH ALREADY!

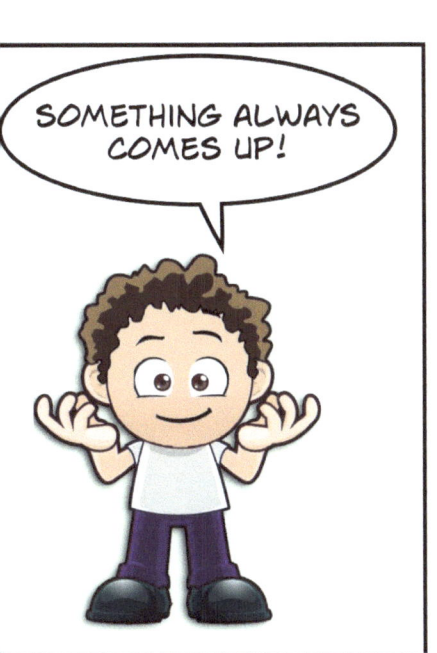

SOMETHING ALWAYS COMES UP!

INNER FIT GIRL SAYS:

FINDING TIME FOR EXERCISE IS HARD WHEN YOU'RE A BUSY BEE.

TRY GETTING UP A LITTLE EARLIER TO FIT YOUR WORKOUT IN. OR DOING SOME KNEE BENDS WHILE YOU ARE ON THE PHONE.

EVERY LITTLE BIT HELPS!

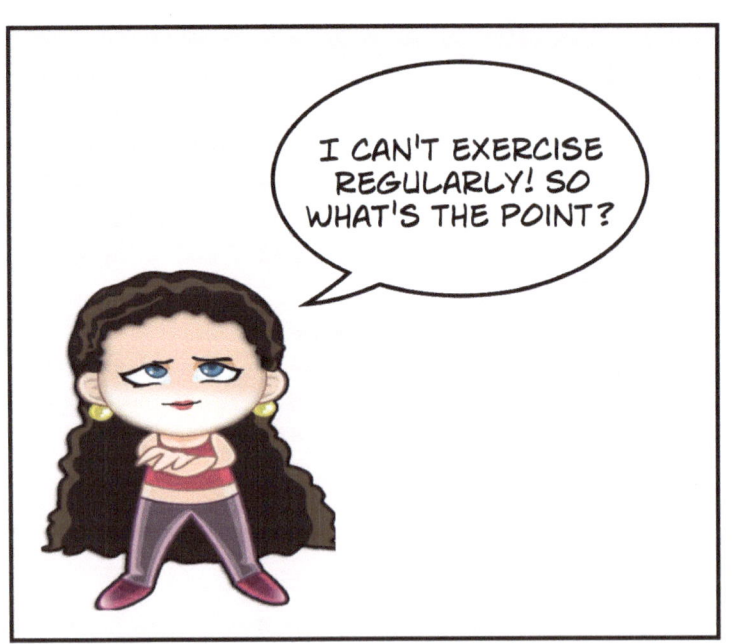

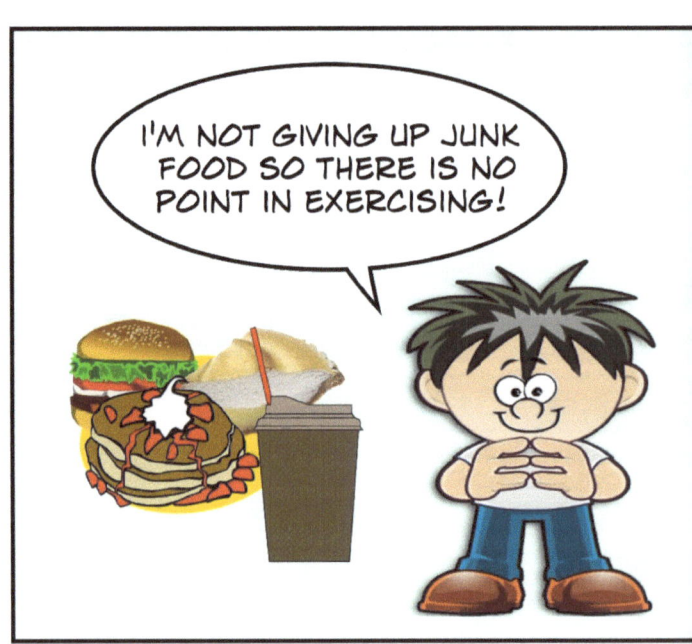

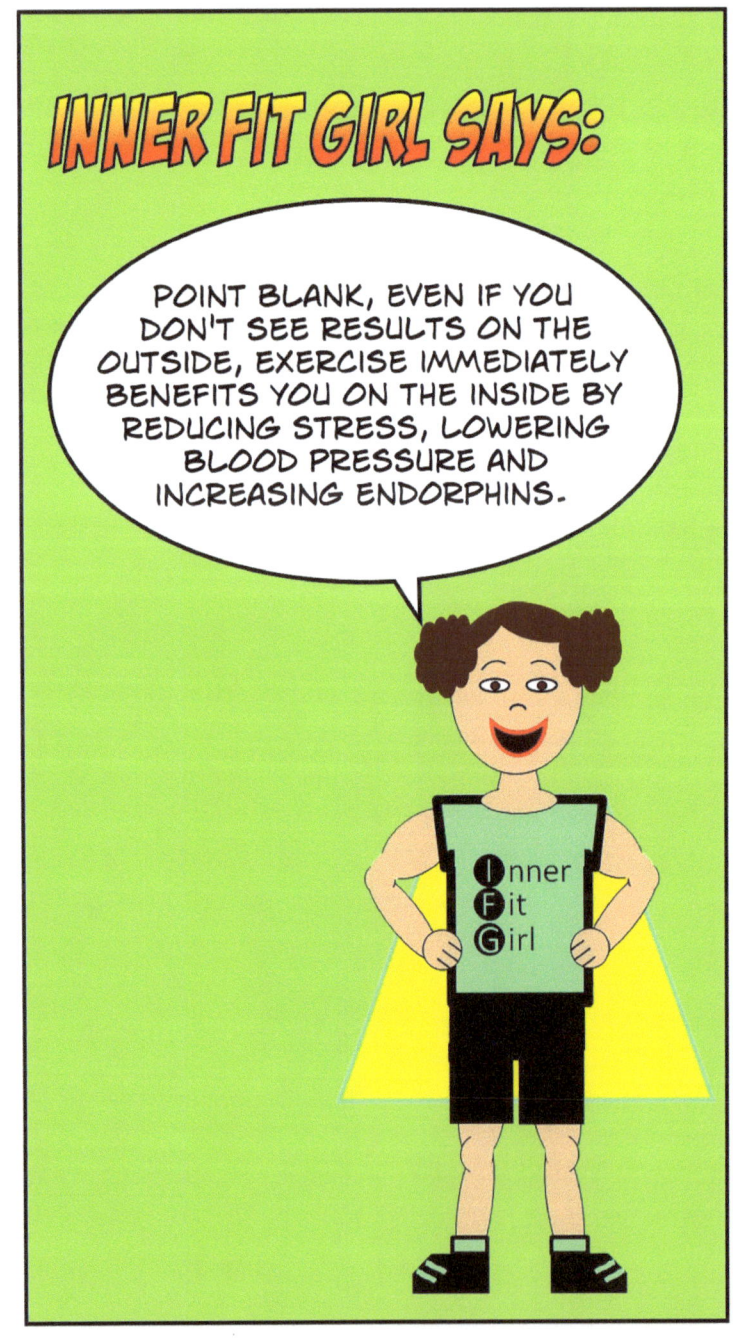

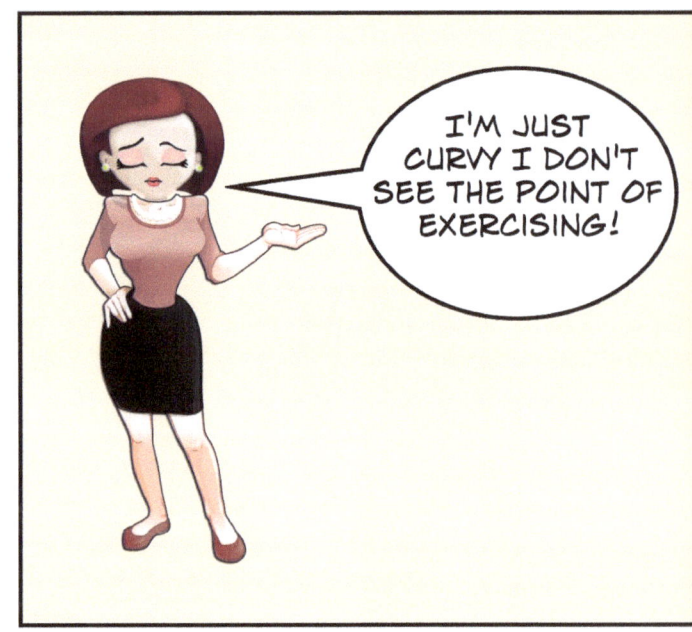

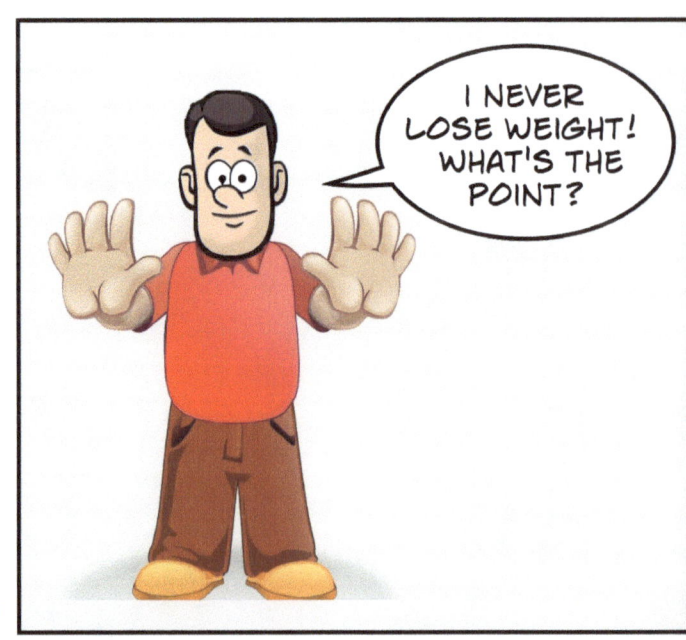

18

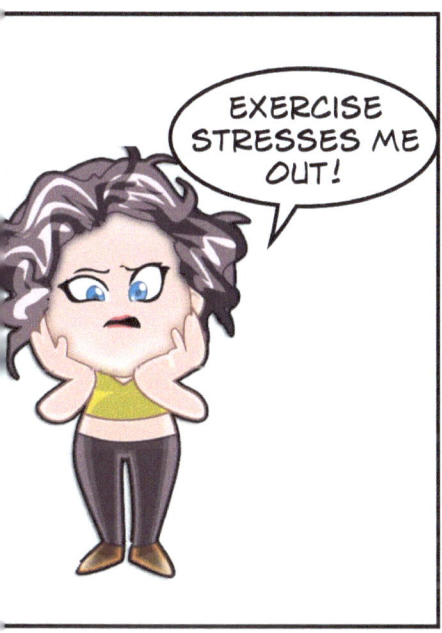

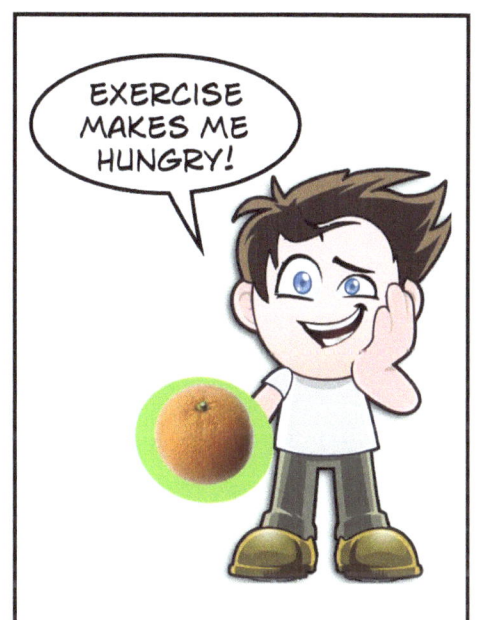

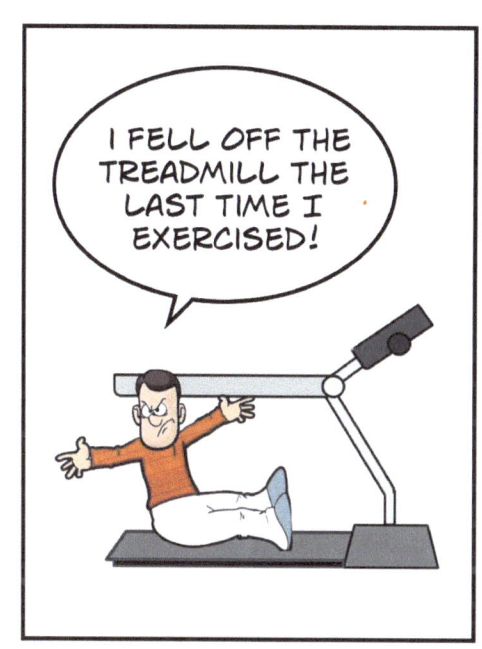

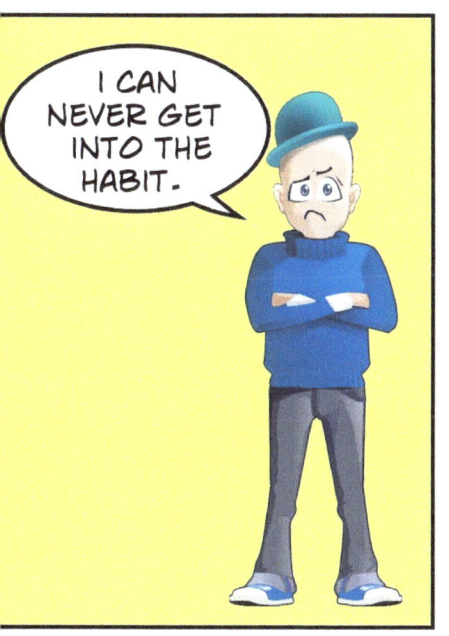

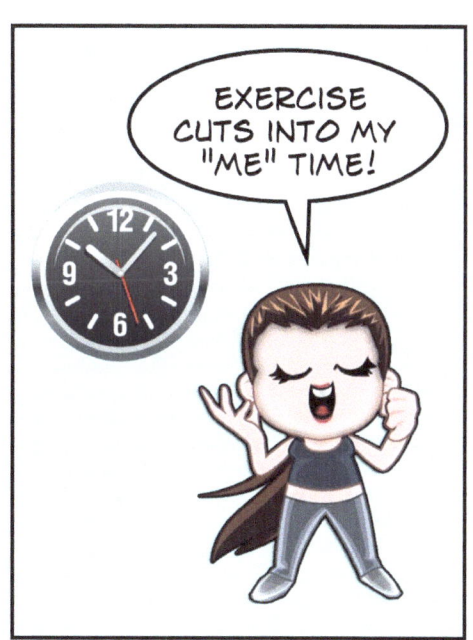

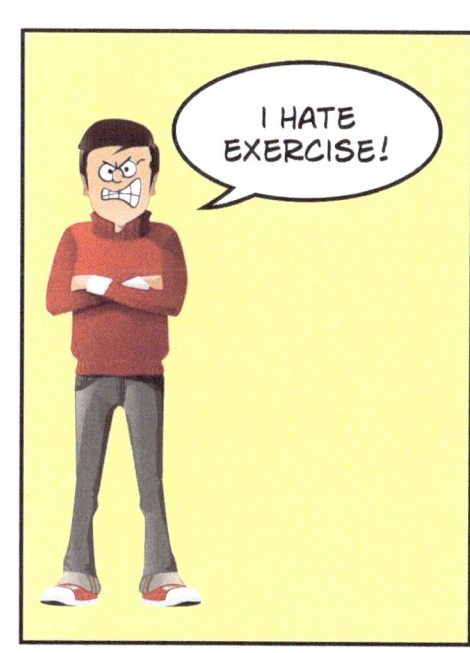

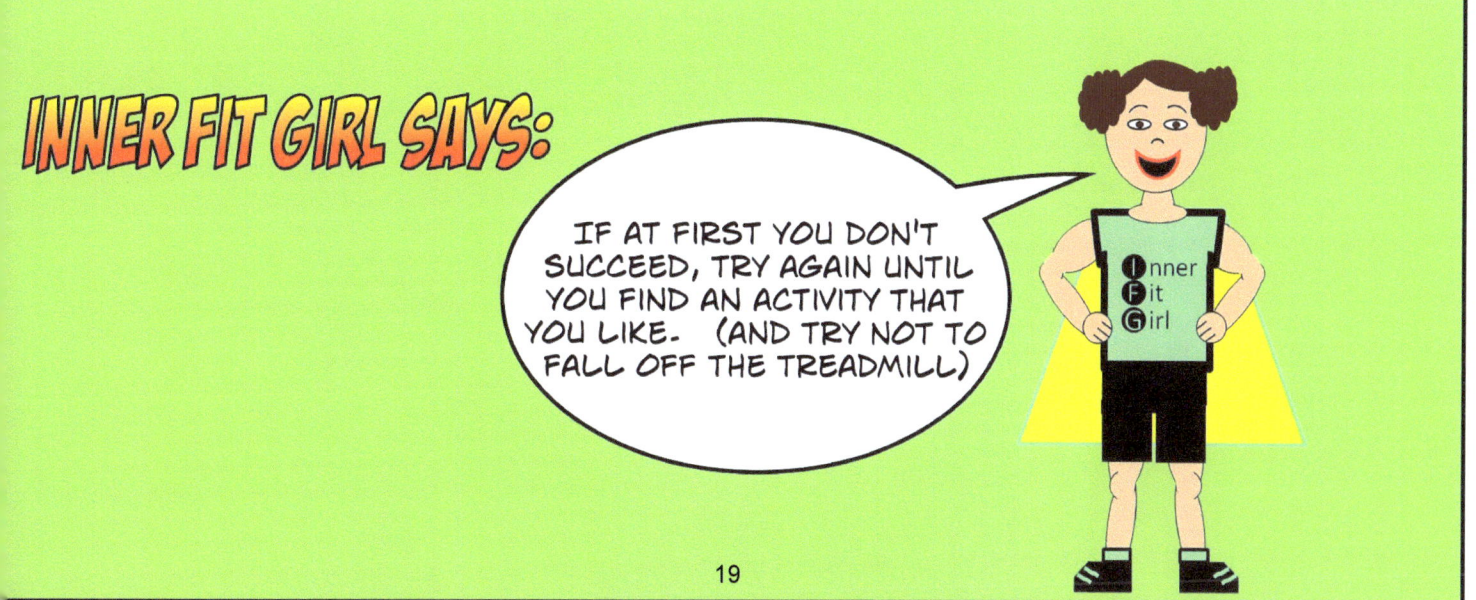

19

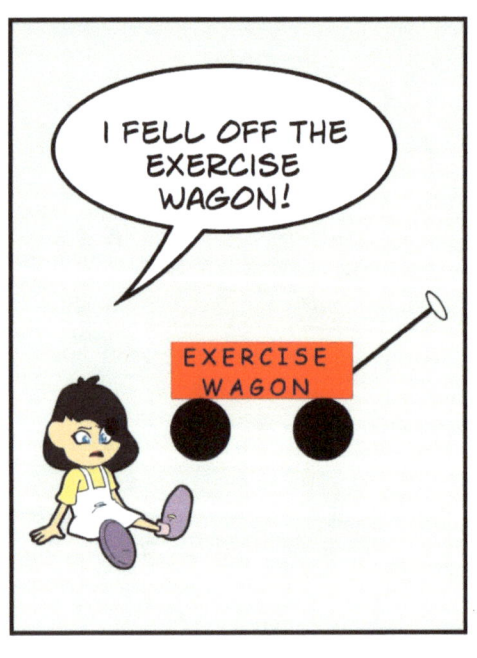

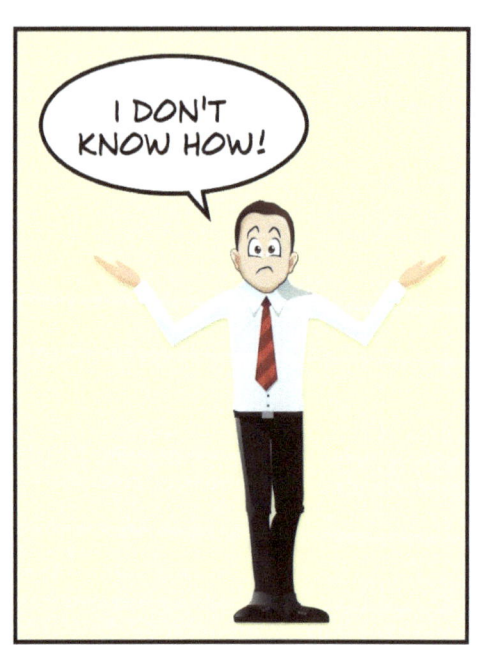

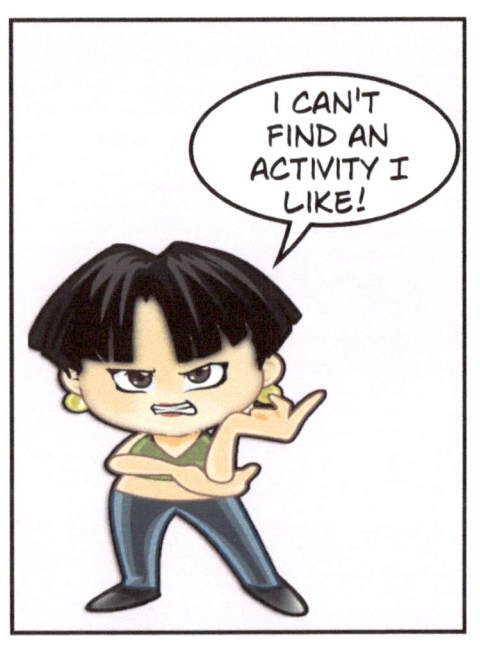

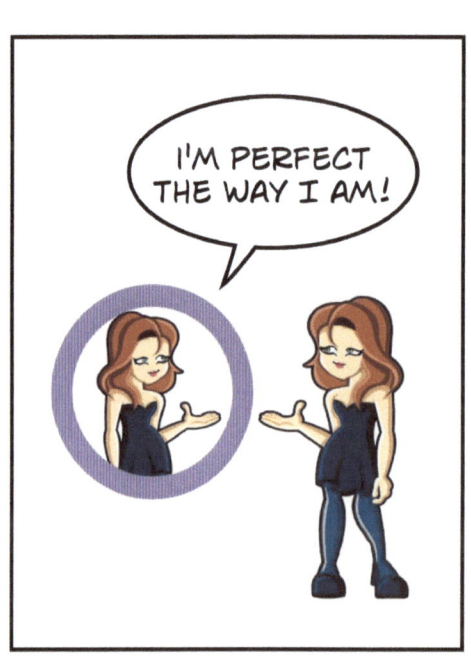

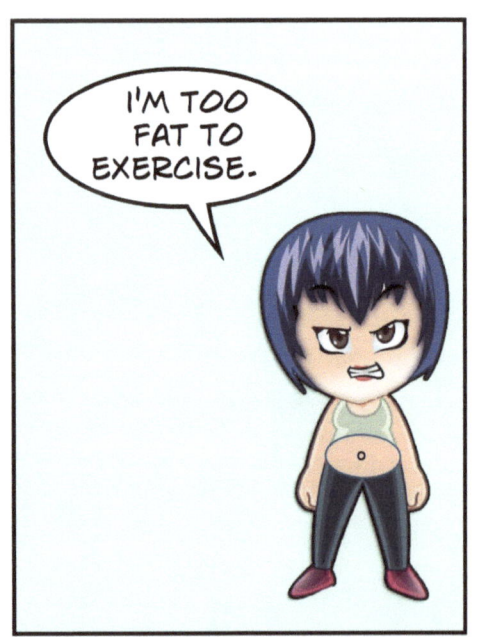

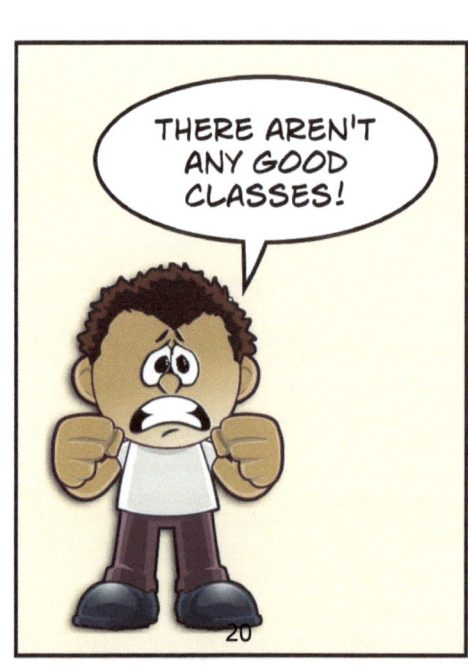

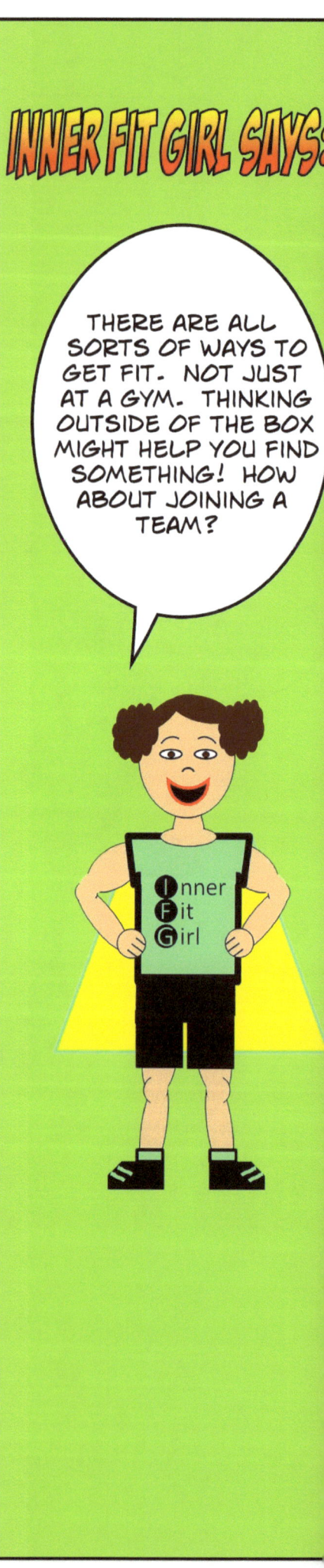

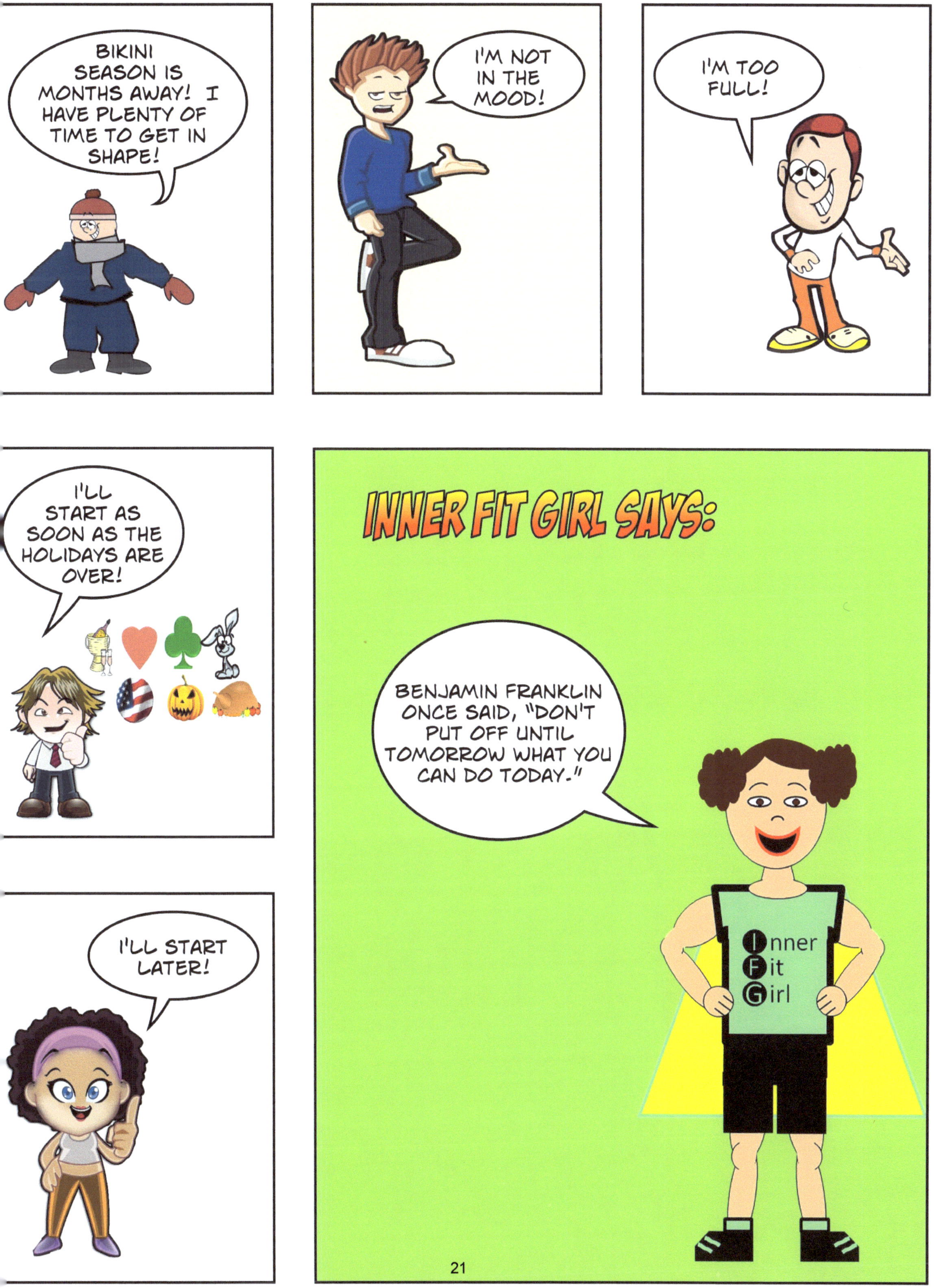

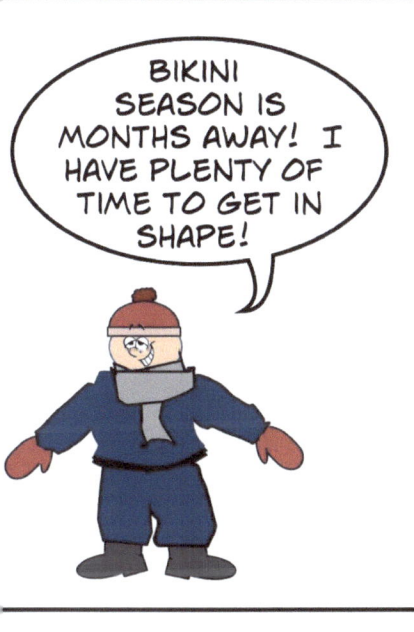

BIKINI SEASON IS MONTHS AWAY! I HAVE PLENTY OF TIME TO GET IN SHAPE!

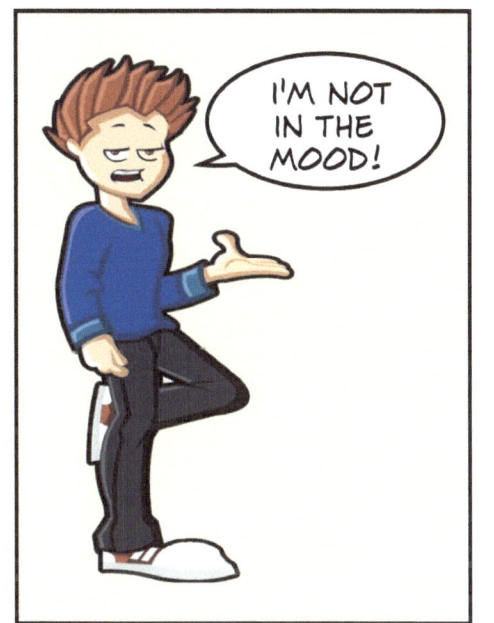

I'M NOT IN THE MOOD!

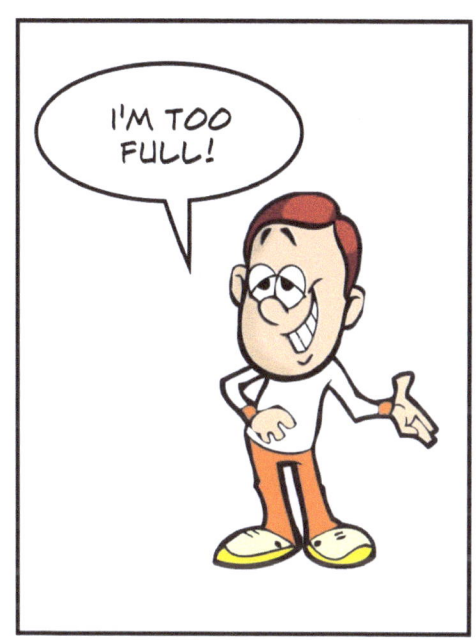

I'M TOO FULL!

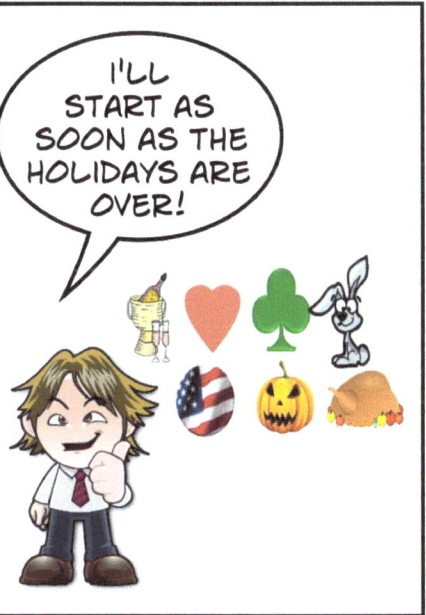

I'LL START AS SOON AS THE HOLIDAYS ARE OVER!

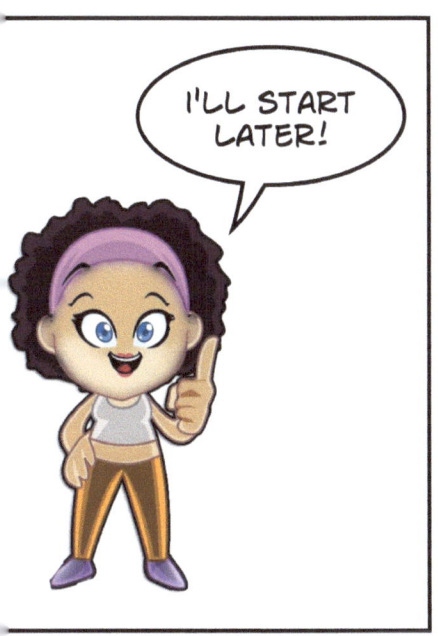

I'LL START LATER!

INNER FIT GIRL SAYS:

BENJAMIN FRANKLIN ONCE SAID, "DON'T PUT OFF UNTIL TOMORROW WHAT YOU CAN DO TODAY."

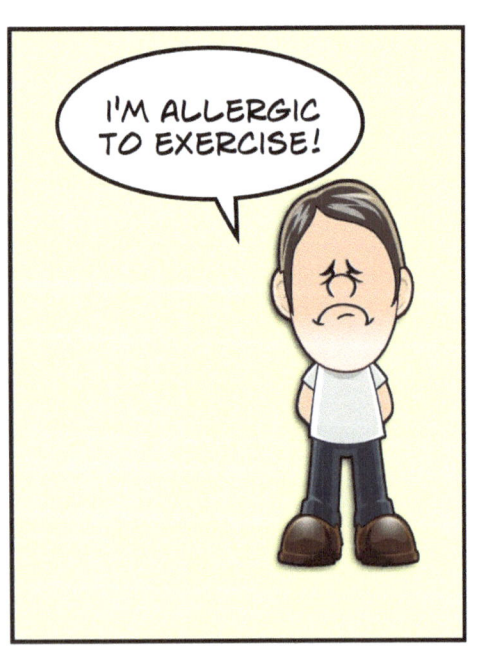

I'M ALLERGIC TO EXERCISE!

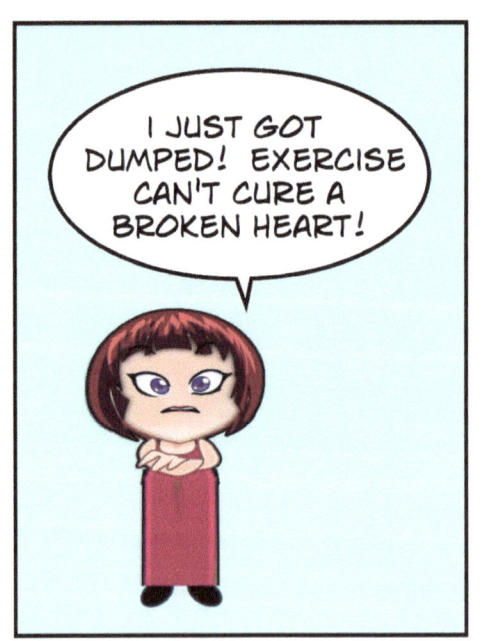

I JUST GOT DUMPED! EXERCISE CAN'T CURE A BROKEN HEART!

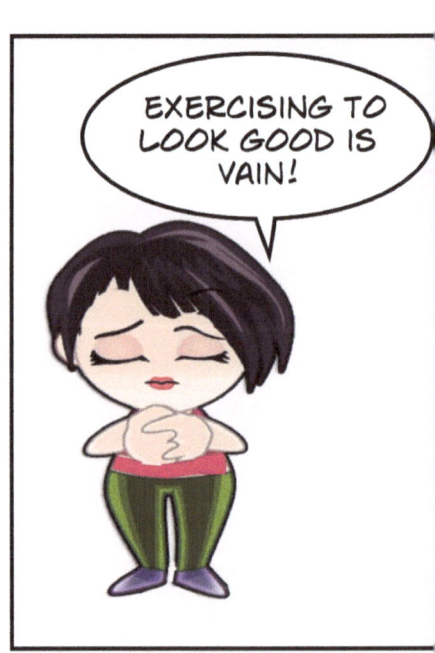

EXERCISING TO LOOK GOOD IS VAIN!

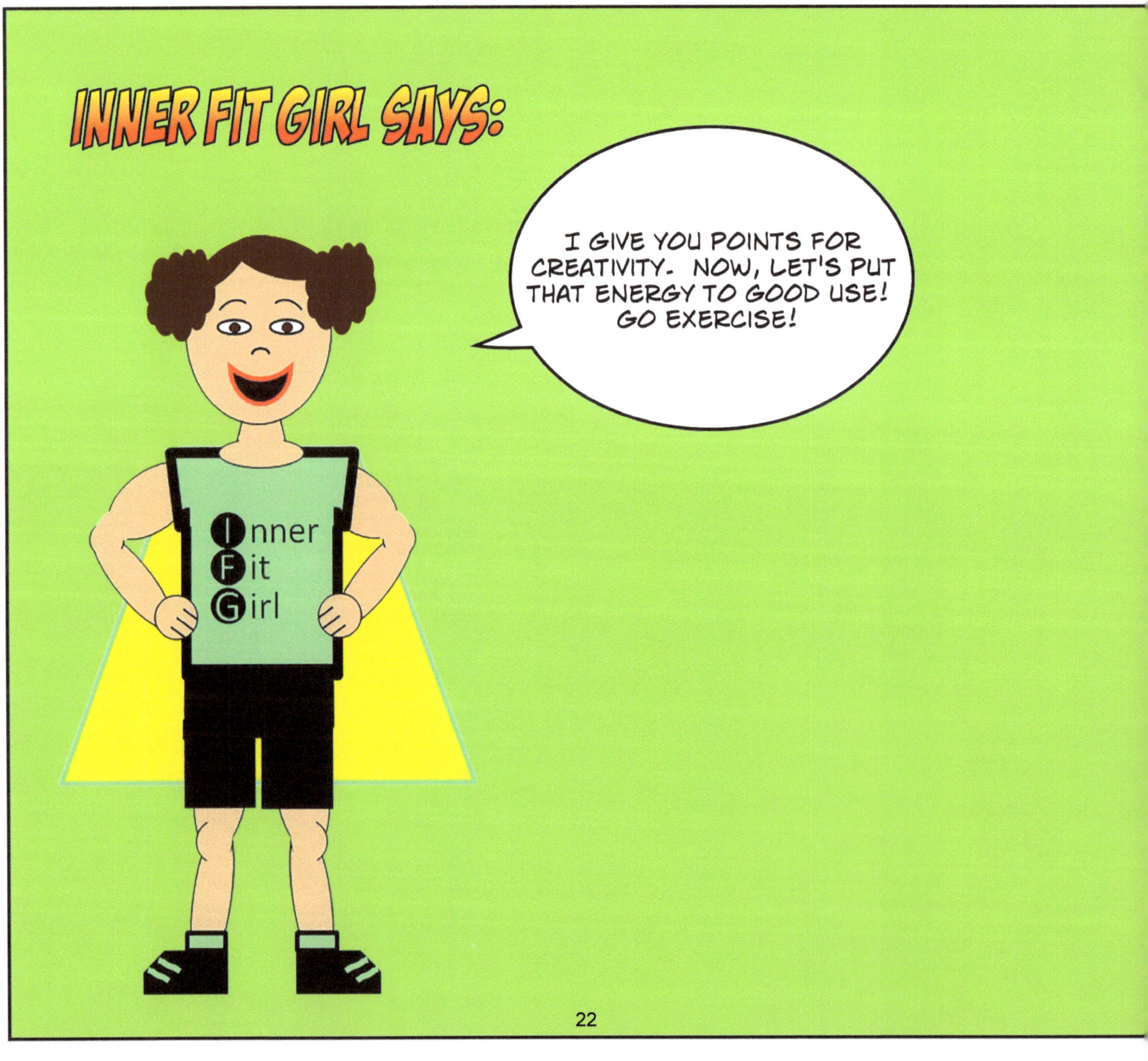

INNER FIT GIRL SAYS:

I GIVE YOU POINTS FOR CREATIVITY. NOW, LET'S PUT THAT ENERGY TO GOOD USE! GO EXERCISE!

Inner
Fit
Girl

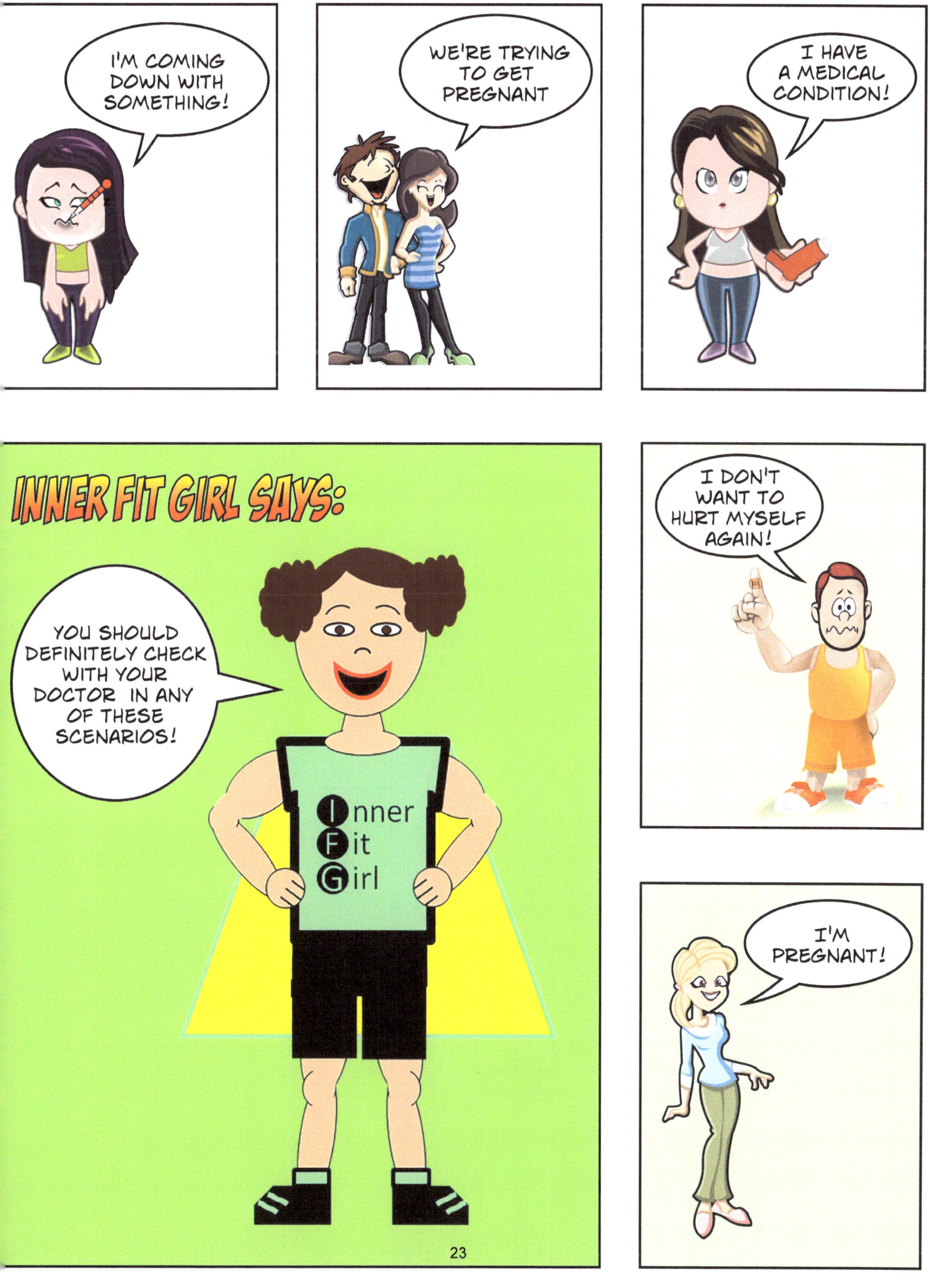

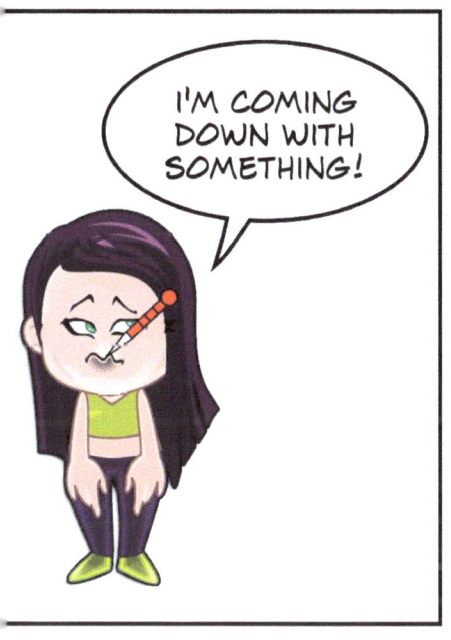

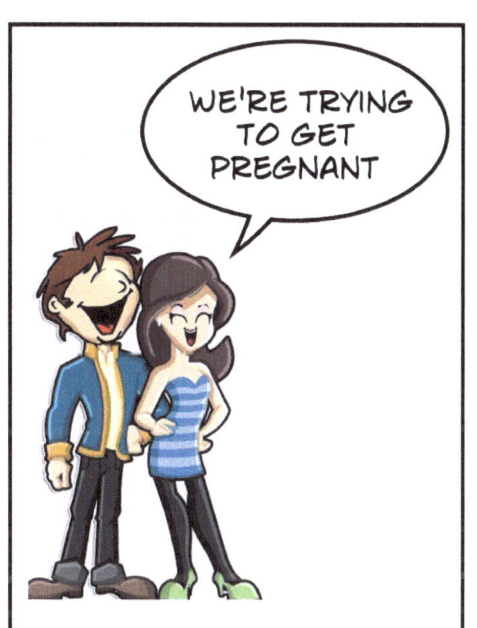

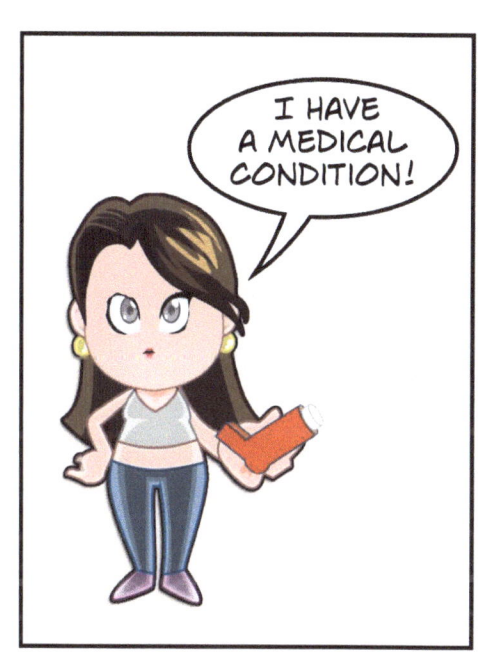

INNER FIT GIRL SAYS:

YOU SHOULD DEFINITELY CHECK WITH YOUR DOCTOR IN ANY OF THESE SCENARIOS!

Inner
Fit
Girl

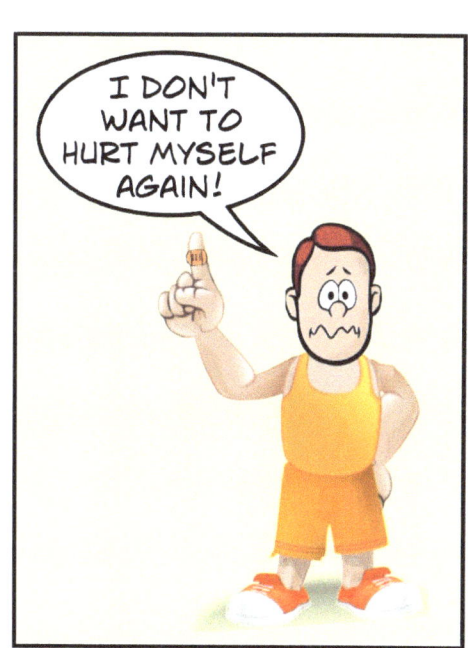

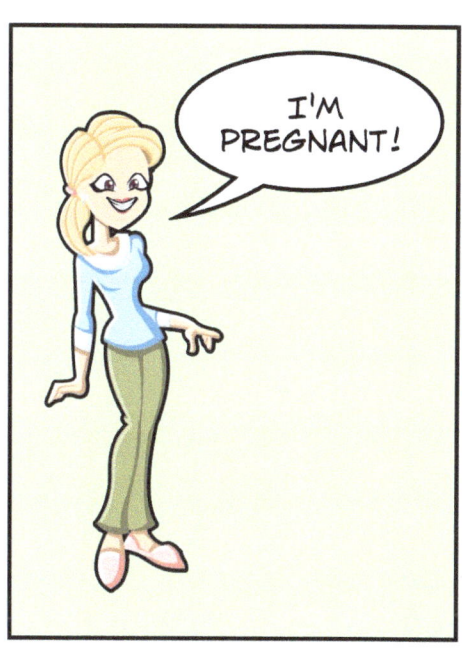

INNER FIT GIRL'S FINAL THOUGHTS

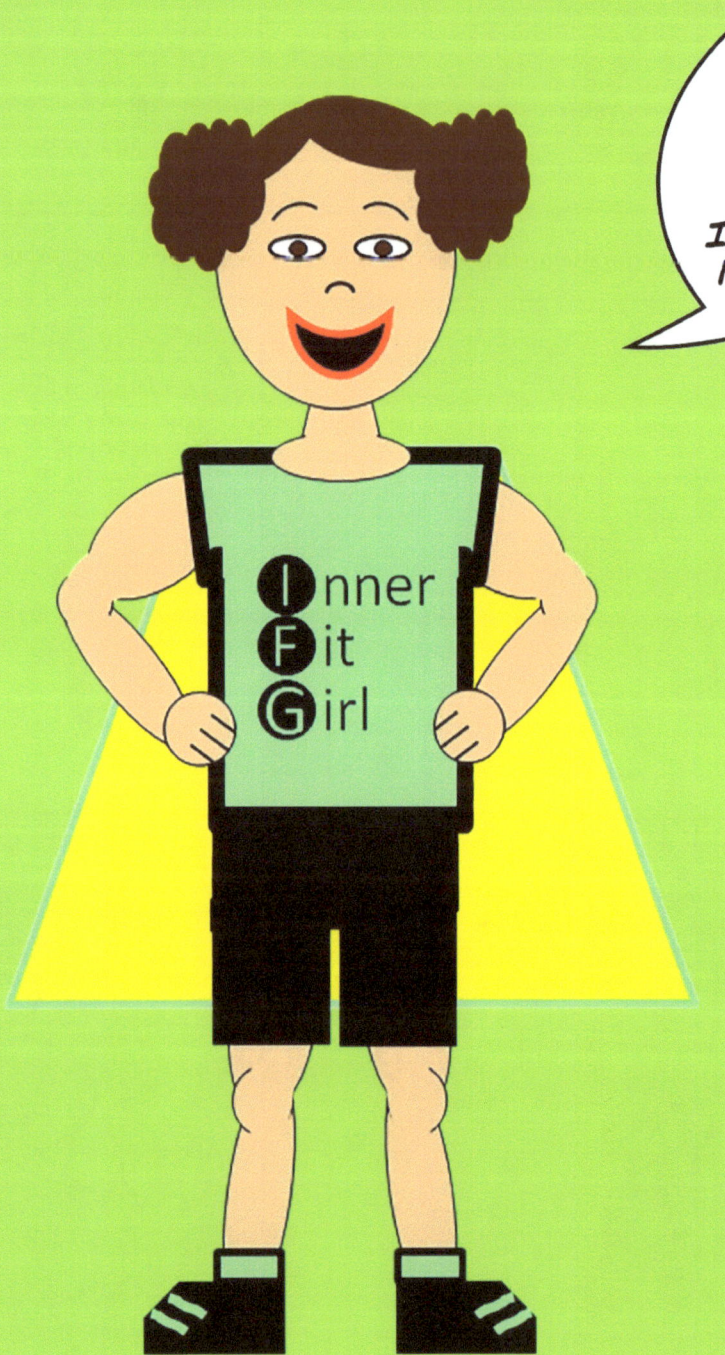

TIRED OF MAKING EXCUSES?

TAKE A WALK!

AND STAY TUNED FOR *INNER FIT GIRL: ADVENTURES IN EXERCISE* TO HELP YOU GET STARTED!!!